MARXISM AND THE SCIENCE OF WAR

MARXISM AND THE SCIENCE OF WAR

EDITED, WITH AN INTRODUCTION,
BY BERNARD SEMMEL

OXFORD UNIVERSITY PRESS
1981

Oxford University Press, Walton Street, Oxford OX2 6DP

OXFORD LONDON GLASGOW
NEW YORK TORONTO MELBOURNE WELLINGTON
KUALA LUMPUR SINGAPORE HONG KONG TOKYO
DELHI BOMBAY CALCUTTA MADRAS KARACHI
NAIROBI DAR ES SALAAM CAPE TOWN

Published in the United States
by Oxford University Press, New York

British Library Cataloguing in Publication Data

Marxism and the science of war.
1. War and society – Addresses, essays, lectures
I. Semmel, Bernard
355'.02 U21.5 80-41151

ISBN 0-19-876112-0
ISBN 0-19-876113-9 Pbk

Set by Graphic Services, Oxford
and printed in Great Britain
at the University Press, Oxford
by Eric Buckley
Printer to the University

IN MEMORY OF T.B.S. AND A.B.

PREFACE

As a historian of ideas who has written on related subjects, I have long been attracted to the study of strategical thought, particularly to the role played by ideology in the shaping of a nation's strategic doctrine. One reason for my turning to the relationship of ideology and strategy is a sense of uneasiness at the failure of Western observers fully to appreciate the considerable part that Marxism plays in Soviet military thinking, or, for that matter, the influence which Western liberalism exerts in producing both the virtues and the disturbing ambiguities which mark our own. In a forthcoming study of British naval strategy in the two centuries before 1914, I hope to explore a part of the historical background of the influence of liberal ideology on strategy. This present volume aims to provide, from the writings and speeches of the chief formulators of Marxist and Marxist-Leninist thought, a view of their absorption with the relationship of Marxism to the science of war. The subject has not received as much attention from students of strategy as it deserves. I do not wish to claim that the influence of ideology is everywhere decisive but rather that ideology, particularly as it affects morale or national psychology, informs every part of a strategic doctrine, and can prove decisive, more particularly in our time than in previous epochs.

Even Marxists have not been much aware of how much intellectual energy the founders of historical materialism gave to military questions. This was more particularly Engels's expertise, but Marx also devoted himself to this study, as did Lenin, Trotsky, and Mao. (Indeed, it was primarily Mao's military writings which led his followers to place him in the pantheon of communist thinkers.) All these writers explored the strategy and tactics necessary to the making of a revolution from the vantage-point of Marxist theory. Their followers and successors, inspired by the successful revolutions in Russia,

China, Cuba, and elsewhere, have extended these efforts to include the global struggle between so-called 'proletarian' and 'capitalist' nations. The relationship between capitalism and war has been explored by a number of Marxist theorists of our century, notably Luxemburg, Bukharin, and Lenin, and it would be difficult to appreciate the thrust of Marxist military doctrine without taking into account what Marxist economics had to say about war. It is only in these terms, moreover, that we can properly understand why the Soviet view of nuclear war appears to differ so profoundly from that of the West.

All these subjects are discussed in the readings included in this volume. It may be useful to stress that this collection does not include the works of men who though perhaps both Marxist-Leninists and writers on military affairs, did not seriously consider the relationship between Marxism and the science of war. Both Stalin and the Vietnamese General Giap, for example, fall into this category.

In my introduction, I have attempted a double analysis: both of how Marxist ideology helped to shape a Marxist science of war, and of how the science of war has altered the face of Marxism. The relevant sections of this introductory essay bear the principal burden in preparing the reader for the study of the documents. Other preparatory information will also be found in the brief remarks preceding the major sections into which the volume is divided.

The decision to produce this collection grew out of a course I initiated at my university a few years ago on 'Modern Strategies of War'. I hope that the readings prove useful not only to those enrolled in similar courses, but also to professional students of strategical doctrines, as well as those general readers with a serious interest in military subjects. In this way, I hope, the volume may make a contribution to the necessary rethinking of the strategical doctrine of the West in the years ahead.

I much appreciate the advice of a number of present and former colleagues who have read and commented on the introductory essay, or with whom I have discussed certain of its conclusions. This group includes Frank E. Myers, Richard T. Rapp, and David F. Trask, as well as my wife Maxine. My wife has typed the manuscript, and she and my son Stuart have helped in the chore of xeroxing the selections. The book is dedicated to the memory of my mother, Tillie Beer Semmel, who died this year, to whose love and indomitable spirit I owe so much. It is dedicated as well to the memory of my uncle, her brother, Aaron Beer, whose persistent challenges taught me something of the strategy of defense, and who first revealed to me the tactics and strategy of baseball on the many Sundays spent in his company at the old New York Polo Grounds.

Bernard Semmel

Stony Brook, NY
November 1979

ACKNOWLEDGEMENTS

The editor and publisher gratefully acknowledge permission to reprint the following copyright material: Nikolai Bukharin: Extracts from *Imperialism and World Economy* (1929). Reprinted by permission of International Publishers, New York. Régis Debray: Extracts from *Revolution in the Revolution?*. Copyright © 1967 by Librairie François Maspero. English Translation Copyright 1967 by Monthly Review Press. Reprinted by permission of Monthly Review Press. Frederick Engels: Extracts from *The Class Struggles in France, 1848–50* (1964). By permission of International Publishers, New York. Extracts from *Anti-Dühring* (1955). By permission of Lawrence & Wishart Ltd., London. S. G. Gorshkov: Extracts from *The Sea Power of the State* (1978). Reprinted by permission of Pergamon Press Ltd., Oxford. S. I. Krupnov: 'According to the laws of dialectics' (trans. Harriet F. Scott) from *The Nuclear Revolution in Soviet Military Affairs* (W. R. Kintner and H. F. Scott, Univ. of Oklahoma Press, 1968). Reprinted by permission of Mrs. Harriet Fast Scott. V. I. Lenin: Extracts from *Imperialism: The Highest Stage of Capitalism* (1939) and *Selected Works* (1967), by permission of International Publishers, New York. Extracts from *Collected Works* (1960–70), by permission of Lawrence & Wishart Ltd., London. Lin Piao: Extracts from 'Long Live the Victory of People's War' in *Strategy for Conquest* (ed. Jay Mallin, 1970). By permission of the University of Miami Press. Rosa Luxemburg: Extracts from 'Militarism as a Province of Accumulation' in *The Accumulation of Capital* (trans. Dr. Agnes Schwarzchild 1951). Reprinted by permission of Routledge & Kegan Paul Ltd. Ernest Mandel: Extracts from *Marxist Economic Theory* (trans. from the French by B. Pearce, n.e. 1972; repr. 1978). Reprinted by permission of The Merlin Press Ltd. Mao Tse-tung: Extracts from *Selected Military Writings* by Chairman Mao Zedong (1966). Reprinted by permission of the Foreign

Languages Press, Peking. Karl Marx: Extracts from *On America and the Civil War* (ed. and trans. S. K. Padover, 1972). Copyright © 1972 by S. K. Padover. Reprinted by permission of McGraw-Hill Book Company. V. D. Sokolovskii: Extracts from *Soviet Military Strategy* (ed. Harriet F. Scott, 1974). Reprinted by permission of Crane, Russak and Company, New York 10017. Leon Trotsky: Extracts from *Military Writings* (trans. John G. Wright et al, 1971). Copyright © 1971. Reprinted by permission of Pathfinder Press, New York.

TABLE OF CONTENTS

INTRODUCTION: MARXISM AND THE SCIENCE OF WAR: THEORY AND PRAXIS

The central concern of Marxism from its earliest days has been, not unnaturally for a political movement, the achievement of power. From the beginning, as well, Marxism has been absorbed with what may be called the 'science of war'—a range of subjects which included all aspects of tactics and strategy. A number of Marxist theorists of the past century and a half have made special studies of military affairs, among them Friedrich Engels who became virtually a professional in the field. These theorists grappled with the relationship between Marxist principles, which Marxists as a matter of philosophical faith regard as affecting a proper understanding of all subjects, and military 'science'. Such a concern was of course to be expected in a movement which prided itself on a carefully reasoned view of historical development, in the light of which both the past and present might be illumined and the future—the inevitable victory of a communist society—foretold.

In the 1840s, Marx and Engels belonged to the group of Left-Hegelians who wished to complete in their own way Hegel's effort to overcome Kant's total separation of pure and practical reason, of knowledge and will—in the terminology they adopted, to unite theory and praxis. (These Left-Hegelians saw the distinction between the two not as a thoroughly antithetic one; they viewed praxis, as infused, in dialectical fashion, with theoretical considerations—with both coexisting in fruitful tension.) From the earliest days of the new philosophy, the Marxists sought not merely to understand the world but to change it: theory would provide an essential guide to a better understanding of the means by which an exploitative and corrupt order might be transformed through human activity (praxis) into an equitable and wholesome one. This tension between theory and practice would be most evident in discussions of the most effective means to achieve power, in efforts to relate Marxism and the science of politics and war. Marx and Engels initially saw in the unfolding events of the 1848 revolution the political and military model for realizing their aspirations. But the finality of defeat brought about a decisive change in their views.

The original heroic view of the Marxist task was submerged for much of the nineteenth century by what many present-day Marxists deride as the crude mechanistic materialism of the Second International. The pre-1914 German Social Democrats, the leading Marxist party of the period, expected an almost automatic triumph to be brought about by the contradictions of the new industrial system, by the increasing misery of the proletariat. They abandoned the romantic, Promethean element so apparent in the 1848 revolution—in which both Marx and Engels had actively participated—as doomed to failure given the strength of the Army in the various bourgeois countries. After the Russian Revolution, and the failure of proletarian revolution in the West, the heroic element was revived in Marxist practice, and has increasingly displaced the earlier emphasis on waiting for the consequences of objective social development. There have been very few twentieth-century Marxists who have permitted theoretical considerations to inhibit actions they thought called for by practical necessities. In the realm of Marxist philosophy, in an effort to unite theory and practice, the Frankfurt School (most prominently Horkheimer, Adorno, and Marcuse) from the 1930s onward has insisted on the importance of restoring the subjective (heroic) element in praxis, following the example of Marx in the 1840s.

Still, Soviet, Chinese, and Cuban generals and political leaders continue to insist, with occasional qualifications, that their over-all view of war, their grand strategy, so to speak, was grounded in traditional Marxist theory. Like Clausewitz, the Prussian general whose book *On War* was much admired by Marx and Engels, as well as by Lenin and Stalin, they see war as the pursuit of politics by other means, and their politics certainly lie within the purview of the Marxist philosophy of international society. For Marxists, the triumph of communism was a matter of historical necessity. It was an open question, however, as to whether this victory were to be accomplished through violent revolution, the ordinary democratic political processes, or, as the twentieth century advanced, through war.

In the 1960s, Marxists of a new sort, inspired by the successes in China and in Cuba of the revival of the heroic method of bringing theory and praxis into harmony, turned traditional Marxism on its head, and formulated a Marxism that would be appropriate for the military strategy they had found to be effective in the struggle to achieve power. In the Soviet Union, an earlier pragmatic posture has given way to one that at times appears to judge weapons systems by the laws of Marxist dialectics, to see war as the instrument for the proletarianization of the exploited classes of the West, and a nuclear confrontation as necessary to the fulfilment of the Marxist ultimate synthesis.

But, while all Marxists would agree on the relevance of dialectical materialism to grand strategy, there has been some controversy in the past century as to whether generals ought to deduce their military methods—their ordinary strategy and their tactics— from Marxist postulates, a question which we shall see was to establish an interesting connection with the larger one. Such a discussion somewhat transformed a dialectical issue to the more conventional one in military circles to which it bears a clear if somewhat crude relationship—whether war was an art or a science, whether its practitioners ought to be empiricists or the followers of a rigid doctrine. In the last century, Engels wrote on both sides of this question. In the first three decades of his absorption with military questions, he had adopted a more or less empirical posture, but then he moved to a more doctrinaire position, grounded on the principles of dialectical materialism.

Engels on War: Art or Science?

The problem of Marxism and the science of war must begin with Marx, and more particularly with Engels, from whose writings both doctrinaires and empiricists derived confirmation of their views. 'I am now reading, among other things, Clausewitz's *On War*,' Engels wrote to Marx in early 1858, finding the work 'an extraordinary way of philosophizing on those matters, but very good.' 'On the question as to whether one ought to speak of the Art of War or the Science of War, his [Clausewitz's] answer is that war is most like Commerce':

'fighting is in war,' Engels continued, describing the Prussian general's view with approval, 'what cash payment is in trade; as seldom as it may in reality need to take place, everything is directed toward it, and in the end it must occur and decide the issue.'[1] What Clausewitz appeared to be saying (and to which Engels implied agreement) was that just as Commerce depended on both the Science of political economy and the Art of bargaining in the market place, so did War depend on both the principles of a military 'science', which generations of writers on strategy and tactics had attempted to discover, and the *Arte della guerra* (the Art, in the sense of craft or guild, of War) of which Machiavelli had written in the sixteenth century.

Machiavelli, Clausewitz, and the early Engels all saw war as a highly skilled profession, like medicine and the law, which although dependent on the knowledge to be secured from a variety of sciences, was at bottom a craft.

There was another tradition that saw war as the application of the principles of a military science: to follow those principles was virtually to ensure victory; to neglect them was to make defeat a certainty. Many of the military writers in the seventeenth and eighteenth centuries had endeavoured to discover the principles of this science. We find evidences of this in the Count de Guibert's *Essai gènèral de tactique*, which he described as 'the science of all times, all places and all arms', a book which made him the lion of the Paris salons of the 1770s. Guibert had distilled his military science from a careful study of the battles of Frederick the Great, who was supposed to have become furious at the Frenchman's revelation of his secrets. A German officer in the wars against Napoleon, Freiherr Dietrich von Bülow, followed a similar scheme in his *Geist des neueren Kriegssystems*, published in 1799. Von Bülow, attempting to account for French successes in the wars that followed the Revolution, stressed the importance of such principles as that which postulated a 'base of operations' from whose ends two 'lines of operation' had to be projected to converge upon the target at minimally a 90° angle. The chief nineteenth-century advocate of this Enlightenment tradition which saw war as a science was the Swiss theorist, Antoine Henri Jomini, who rose to become Marshal Ney's chief of staff. (In 1813, Jomini, despairing of promotion beyond the rank of Brigadier-General, deserted to the Russian Army.)

Jomini, like von Bülow, also attempted to distil his military science from a careful study of the battles of both Frederick and Napoleon. While critical of von Bülow's 'trigonometric' rationalism, Jomini appeared even more unhappy with Clausewitz's 'skepticism in matters of military science'. Certainly, the early volumes of his *Traité des grandes opérations militaires*, begun in 1804, and his two-volume *Précis de l'art de la guerre*, of 1838, saw war as science, and not art, as the title of the later volume would suggest. 'There have existed in all times, fundamental principles, on which depend good results in warfare,' he wrote in his 1804 work; 'those principles are unchanging, independent of the kind of weapons, of historical time and of place.' Like von Bülow, he emphasized the concept of the base of operations, and added such additional principles as the necessity of gaining control of at least three sides of a rectangular 'zone of operations' (which he described in a precise geometric fashion), the superiority of interior to exterior lines when a double line of operations was employed, and the overwhelming importance of the principle of concentrating one's forces. Jomini's writings were taken up with alacrity by military academies throughout the world. It has been said that the generals of both sides of the American Civil War carried translations of Jomini in their knapsacks and referred to his prescriptions on the eve of battle.[2]

Engels was much taken with Jomini, whose works he had studied with care, as well as with Clausewitz.[3] Marx does not appear to have read the more technical writings of Jomini, but he did read Clausewitz in the course of some writing on military questions upon which he was engaged (of which more later). Concerning Clausewitz, Marx wrote that 'the chap has a common sense that borders on brilliance'.[4] We might note that Clausewitz's 'skepticism' concerning geometrical military theory was accompanied by a conviction that *emotion* played a critical role in war. Much of his strategic doctrine, indeed, was derived from this essentially Romantic–*Sturm und Drang*–view of warfare.

While both Marx and Engels read extensively in military

history and theory, it was Engels who, as we have noted, made the field his special concern from the time of his participation in the revolutionary fighting in Baden in 1848. During the revolutionary days of that year and the one following, when the Hungarians under the leadership of Kossuth rose up against the Austrian monarchy in an effort to achieve independence, Engels watched what was happening in the Habsburg domains with the keenest interest, convinced that Kossuth's success in Hungary would make a German revolution more likely. Following the day-to-day events of the war in Hungary, he became fascinated by military questions. The failure of the Hungarian rebels convinced him of the 'colossal importance' of the 'military branch' if there were to be a successful revolution. (Towards the end of his life, he was persuaded that the proletarian revolution might be a by-product of an international war.) In the years following 1848, Engels turned his energies to the mastering of all the divisions of military science. This was to be his own special field, supplementing Marx's expertise on economic matters. Just as Marx was known by the nickname of Mohr, because of his dark Moorish complexion (although one may speculate, perhaps more romantically than correctly, that this may have been a variation of the name of the hero of Schiller's *Die Räuber*, Karl von Moor, with whom Marx had strongly identified in his early years), Engels was called the General. (Our subject may be seen as a charting of the relationship between 'the General' and Marx as 'the Economist'.) In 1851, Engels turned to Joseph Weydemeyer, a former Prussian artillery officer who had fought for the revolutionary cause in 1848, and who was later to emigrate to America and to serve as a Colonel in the Northern Army during the Civil War Weydemeyer provided him with the books he would need to acquire expertise on military questions, and became Engels's particular confidant on the progress of his military studies.

Engels had an additional reason at this time for wishing to master military science. During the fighting in Baden in 1848, Engels had briefly served as aide-de-camp to August von Willich, a former Prussian lieutenant who, because of his socialist views, had defected to the Volunteer Army of Baden and the Palatinate, and had fought against the Prussian regulars.

In 1850, Willich was a member, along with Marx and Engels, of the Communist League, composed primarily of Germans in London who had fled the defeat of the revolution in their homeland. In alliance with a group of *émigré* Prussian officers, and much to the opposition, and, indeed, disgust of Marx and Engels, Willich put himself forward to the League as the leader of a military *putsch* that would make him the master of Germany. Marx and Engels were offended at the bluster with which Willich presented his views in the London public houses catering for the German *émigrés*. This was hardly a proper approach to social revolution, in the view of the fathers of scientific socialism, particularly after the disappointing experiences of 1848. Moreover, Marx and Engels had no use for Willich personally, thinking him an able enough leader of a regiment of volunteers, but hardly the general of an army. Engels apparently devoted himself with even greater energy to military affairs so as to prove to this 'military gang' of ex-officers that 'at least one of the civilians' who opposed their views could argue with them on a professional level. (Willich also was to emigrate to the United States, in 1853, where he became editor of the German-language *Cincinnati Republikaner*, continuing to oppose Marx's and Engels's views among *émigré* German socialists; with the coming of the Civil War, he was to become first a Colonel and then a Brigadier-General of Ohio contingents in the Union Army.)[5]

Engels's studies were apparently thorough and systematic.[6] Very soon, we find him supplying Marx with articles on military subjects which appeared under Marx's name in the *New York Daily Tribune*. For the *Tribune*, Engels wrote on the Crimean War, the Indian Mutiny, and the Spanish war in Morocco, among other subjects. When the American Civil War terminated the connection with the *Tribune*, the Viennese paper, *Die Presse*, published Engels's analyses of the fighting between the Union and the Confederacy. Engels attempted to secure a post as writer upon military affairs with the *London Daily News* in 1854, but was not successful.[7] In the early 1860s, he managed a connection with the *Volunteer Journal*, an organ of the movement for a volunteer militia that swept England in 1859, for which he wrote articles on the Volunteers and on the history of the Rifle. He also established a brief relationship with the *Manchester Guardian*, to which he supplied, in 1866, his military analyses of the Seven Weeks' War between Austria and Prussia.

Engels's and Marx's most extensive writings on military subjects were for the *New American Cyclopaedia*, which their long-time friend and one of the editors of the *Tribune*, Charles A. Dana, was editing in New York on behalf of the *Tribune*. The preparation of these pieces absorbed both of them for a good part of the years of 1857 and 1858, and more sporadically in the two following years.[8] Engels did most of the research and writing, not merely because this had become his primary field of concern, but also so as to leave Marx time for his economic studies. While Marx wrote biographies of the Napoleonic Marshals, and, in collaboration with Engels, on Prussian Field Marshal von Blücher, Engels supplied technical essays on great battles, on weapons such as the arquebus, the bayonet, the bomb, and the catapult, as well as on more general subjects such as the campaign, the cavalry, and the fleet. In two of his articles—on the Army and on the Infantry—Engels was able to display his vast erudition on the subject of war, and to set forth a historical view of the development of military science over the centuries.

What is most noteworthy concerning these essays—which are today much prized as prime examples of Marxist thinking on military subjects in both East Germany and Soviet Russia[9]—is how little of a specifically 'Marxist' character they possess. Moreover, this apparent reluctance to employ a Marxist analysis extended to *all* Engels's military writings of the almost three decades before the publication of the *Anti-Dühring* in 1878. In the sixteen-thousand word article on 'Army', for example, we find a careful and detailed exposition of almost every aspect of the subject—the raising, training, and equipping of armies, their formations and tactics, etc., but very little—except for some conventional discussion of the influence of gunpowder on the break-up of feudalism—concerning the political and social context which even a non-Marxist historian, at that time as now, would find obligatory. The shorter, nine-thousand word article on 'Infantry' was perhaps, but just barely, the more 'Marxist' of the two.[10] Did Engels suppress his views because they were to appear in a bourgeois encyclopaedia? But bourgeois historians like Guizot or Buckle were prepared to provide such sociological underpinnings for their analyses, and their efforts were welcomed by the public, free as such explanations were at that time of any identification with revolutionary socialism. Nor was it a question of insufficient space, for Engels permitted himself to speculate freely on other questions: for example, following Clausewitz, he ventured to predict, inaccurately as it turned out, that 'we shall most likely never see such an army again united for one operation' as the 450,000 Napoleon had mustered for the invasion of Russia in 1812.[11] (There was no effort to anticipate, in this matter, the *Anti-Dühring*'s later insistence that the forms of war would change with the growing importance of the proletariat.) Did Engels, at this time, believe that historical materialism had no application to the study of military subjects? This is a possible explanation, and worth exploring.

But some twenty years later, in 1878, Engels was to adopt an altogether different approach to military science in his *Anti-Dühring*. Engels wrote his lengthy critique of Eugen Karl Dühring at the request of German Marxists, fearful that the new 'socialism' of this philosopher and economist was making inroads upon the rank-and-file of German Social Democracy. Dühring had created a 'system'. In his polemic, Engels found himself outlining a counter-system. In a section on political economy, Engels discussed Dühring's 'force theory', the view that political relationships based on 'direct political force' were the elemental core of historic development, and that economic relationships were merely secondary. Dühring had presented his view in terms of Robinson Crusoe enslaving Friday, while Engels insisted that this enslavement had as its object Friday's production of surplus value for Crusoe's benefit. Here, Engels felt compelled to present a more systematic Marxist view of militarism. He observed that 'nothing is more dependent on economic prerequisites than precisely the army and navy.' Armaments and army organization, strategy and tactics were all the creatures of the stage of economic development not the '"free creations of the mind" of generals of genius'. Engels placed not merely his emphasis, but the entire burden of his argument upon such revolutionary developments as gunpowder and firearms, and the effects upon tactics of such movements as the American and French Revolutions. Such a view of militarism, Engels concluded, was all the more important lest the contemporary bourgeoisie, suffering from Dühring's 'delusion' that force might save their collapsing economy, should imagine that the economic consequences of the steam-engine ... of world trade and the banking and credit developments of the present day, can be blown out of existence by them with Krupp guns and Mauser rifles.' The processes of social evolution, and hence proletarian victory, could not be halted by bourgeois control of armies and armaments.[12]

Engels's earlier military writings, we have suggested, had given evidence of a different and, indeed, contradictory tone. But more than 'tone' was at issue. One or two specific examples of such evident contradictions may be useful. In his article on 'Infantry', for instance, Engels had been ready to describe Frederick the Great's adoption of a military invention of the fourth century BC Theban general Epaminondas as essential to his military success, apparently disregarding the respective stages of economic development in which these two generals flourished. 'Epaminondas was the first to discover the great tactical principle which up to the present day decides almost all pitched battles: the unequal distribution of the troops on the line of the front, in order to concentrate the main attack on one decisive point.' Some pages subsequently in this article, Engels endeavoured to explain the 'mystery' of how Frederick, with resources more limited than those possessed by nineteenth-century Sardinia, could 'carry on a war against almost all Europe'. Frederick—that 'man of genius'—'applied to the line order of battle the system of oblique attack invented by Epaminondas.'[13] In the *Anti-Dühring*, as we have noted, strategy and tactics were described as determined entirely by economic development and were not 'the "free creations of the mind" of generals of genius'. Frederick's adoption of this tactic of Epaminondas was briefly dismissed in the 1878 work as possessing only minor import, Engels noting that 'at the very most, either of the two wings might move forward or keep back a little.'[14] So much then, in his doctrinaire work, for the adoption of the invention of the Theban general by means of which the Prussian 'genius', as he had written twenty years earlier, had successfully waged 'war against almost all Europe'—a subject to which he had devoted nearly a column and a half in his encyclopaedia article.

In the *Anti-Dühring*, to cite another example, Engels was to observe that Prussia's equipment of its infantry with the rifled breech-loader had been a decisive factor in its successful war against Austria in 1866.[15] This was a view consistent with the economic interpretation, and, indeed, was one commonly held by both military specialists and laymen at the time. In his *Manchester Guardian* articles of 1866, however, Engels had dealt very differently, some would say in less simplistic terms, with the war. At the start of hostilities, Engels had predicted an Austrian victory 'in spite of the needle gun' [one form of rifled breech-loaders] possessed by the Prussians, and even despite the fact that, due to grave deficiencies in the Austrian commissariat, the Prussian soldier was likely to be better fed than his Austrian counterpart. Austria would triumph, Engels declared, because of 'superior leadership, organization, tactical formation, and *morale*'. In this, he was perhaps writing as a Clausewitzian, not as an economic determinist. When, none the less, the war went in Prussia's favour, Engels was prepared to assign some importance to the needle gun, but only because the morale of the Prussian soldier, hopeful of achieving German unification, had been greater than Engels had anticipated.[16] Clearly morale and leadership were held to be able to overcome what an economic interpretation must regard as decisive components: a full stomach and an advanced technology.

How, then, can we account for Engels's failure to employ a 'Marxist' method in his earlier military writings? The tone of the military essays written before 1878 bore the marks of the 1840s, the years of 'the General'. Hence the stress upon the subjective, human element in the praxis, the insistence on the importance of morale, leadership, and genius as overriding factors. All this was before Marx and Engels found themselves at the head of a considerable political movement, one that placed its hopes on the despair of the masses, growing out of the contradictions of the capitalist economy, and in bringing about communism by electoral means. The elaboration of a monistic economic interpretation, made necessary by the comprehension of proletarian military helplessness and by the need of the German Social-Democratic leadership to make theory and practice somewhat more harmonious, was the spur to the system-making of the 1878 tract. (Marx proved somewhat more resistant to the introduction of such rigidities by some of his followers. It was to be in response to a continental comrade that he made his celebrated statement—'*Je ne suis pas Marxiste*'.)

There may have been an additional factor in Engels's reluctance to adopt a crude, materialistic approach to military affairs. Since he had devoted himself most particularly to acquiring an expertise in this field, a doctrinaire analysis would have seemed especially unsatisfactory, if only because such a one-sided interpretation would be immediately vitiated by the number of counter-examples that would come easily to his mind. There is, after all, a tendency for specialists to be more indulgent of simplistic formulations in fields other than their own. But there were to be enough doctrinaire Marxists in the decades ahead, prepared to encase military strategy and tactics into Marxist categories, and to determine the validity of any proposition on the basis of its conformity to economic materialism—all this in the systematizing spirit of Guibert, von Bülow, and of the Engels of the *Anti-Dühring*. These doctrinaires adhered to their faith in the undeniable reality of an ultimate Marxist military science even as they struggled to discover its principles. Of course, there continued to be Marxists who took the pragmatic position of Machiavelli, Clausewitz, and the early Engels. Repeatedly, in the course of this century, as we shall see, the differences between Engels's earlier pragmatic views and those of the *Anti-Dühring* became the grounds of intense, and at times violent, conflict among Marxists. But, we must remember, even these Marxist military pragmatists saw their politics, of which war was an extension, in the class terms of dialectical materialism. All these controversies were conducted in the context of a view of economic and political development upon which all could more or less agree. In the analysis of capitalism mounted by twentieth-century Marxists, war always played a central role.

Capitalism, Socialism, and War

In the course of his chapter on military questions in the *Anti-Dühring*, Engels described the naval race, then just beginning, which was to mark the generations before 1914: 'In this competitive struggle between armour-plating and guns, the warship is being developed to a pitch of perfection which is making it both outrageously costly and unuseable in war'. Engels had in mind the development of the self-propelled torpedo which would make 'the smallest torpedo boat . . . superior to the most powerful armoured warship.' Engels was convinced that the enormous costliness of the new warships would keep the bourgeois states from exposing them to threats of destruction. Such an opinion conformed with the theory of savings of the orthodox political economists, with which Marx and Engels agreed; the orthodox theorists rejected the heretical view, long-held by Malthus and his followers, that wasteful consumption was a necessary remedy for the inescapable glut of overproduction. The 'competitive struggle between armour-plating and guns', Engels continued, 'makes manifest also in the sphere of naval warfare those inherent dialectical laws of motion on the basis of which militarism, like every other historical phenomenon, is being brought to its doom in consequence of its own development.' Engels's conclusion, therefore, was that, in accordance with the laws of Marxist dialectics—with thesis being nullified by its antithesis, even as they joined in forming a synthesis, which in turn became a new thesis—militarism, like bourgeois society, was negating itself.[17] This was an entirely appropriate conclusion, perhaps, for a philosophy that could perceive war only in rational, economic terms.

In another generation, when Engels's prediction had proved faulty, Marxists would insist, having revived heretical underconsumptionist economic theories, that capitalism, indeed, required huge military expenditures to overcome its economic contradictions, that, in fact, capitalism could not survive without war. In 1913, the Polish-German Marxist, Rosa Luxemburg wrote in her *Accumulation of Capital* that only by the production of armaments could the surplus portion of the capitalist's income (which if unconsumed would disastrously clog the arteries of the circulation of wealth) be restored to the economy—this by way of wages to workers in the armaments and munitions industries. Her economic analysis, as she made clear, was founded on views of unproductive expenditure similar to those espoused by the Physiocrats, Malthus, and, in particular, the Russian populist and anti-capitalist economist, Vorontsov. But while Vorontsov saw militarism as one of a number of ways in which this surplus profit of the capitalists could re-enter the economy without causing dislocations, and the capitalist as bearing the prime burden for armaments, Luxemburg viewed militarism as absolutely essential to the workings of capitalism, with the financial burden for armaments falling, by way of indirect taxation, entirely on the working class.[18]

The necessity of militarism to the proper functioning of capitalism became an essential of Marxist argument in the twentieth century, usually linked, as it had been by Luxemburg, by the necessity of armaments and war as 'a weapon in the competitive struggle between capitalist countries for areas of non-capitalist civilisation,' that is, imperialism. Rudolf Hilferding's *Finanzkapital*, the first rigorous Marxist analysis of imperialism, published in 1910, had depicted a capitalism which had moved from a stage of free competition to one in which the large banking houses exercised a monopolistic control over industry. Following the argument put forward earlier in the decade by the English liberal economist J. A. Hobson, Hilferding depicted a capitalism forced on to a course of imperial expansion and war because of its need for new markets for its surplus production and new opportunities for its surplus capital. In 1915, Nikolai Bukharin, a leading Bolshevik theoretician, wrote his *Imperialism and World Economy*, which, following Hilferding and other German and Austrian neo-Marxist writings, also depicted imperialism as an inevitable accompaniment of the hegemony of finance capital, which, he declared, 'implies both imperialism and militarism'. 'Capitalist society', he concluded, 'is unthinkable without armaments, as it is unthinkable without wars.' Lenin, in his introduction to Bukharin's work, announced that the '"peaceful" capitalism' of the nineteenth century—the capitalism that Engels had no doubt in mind when he made his dialectical analysis prophesying the end of militarism—had been 'replaced by unpeaceful, militant, catastrophic imperialism.'[19]

Two years later, in 1917, Lenin was to publish his own tract on *Imperialism*, which was to become one of the most influential political works of the twentieth century. One of Lenin's purposes in publishing the essay was to refute Karl Kautsky, the leading German Marxist theorist, who had written of an initially aggressive imperialism evolving into a pacific, and, indeed, even beneficent 'ultra-imperialism', a prediction that suggested that capitalism would resolve its most pressing contradictions—and would, perhaps like Engels's 1878 view of militarism, dialectically negate its aggressive posture. Lenin dismissed such an analysis as un-Marxist, bourgeois reformism. Basing his own views largely on the analysis of Hilferding and Hobson, Lenin saw the new control of both the state and industry by the financiers as having brought capitalism to a repressive and violent stage. In search of a higher rate of profit than that obtainable at home, capitalists were aggressively dividing the as yet undeveloped world so that they might exploit its cheap native labour and plentiful resources. There would always be powers which would feel cheated, and they would always seek new apportionments. This would mean continual wars. By its very nature, capitalism could do nothing to break its dependence on imperialism, and its necessary companions—militarism and war. (Later Marxist economists, including such recent writers as Sweezy, Baran, and Mandel, have not departed from the essentials of Lenin's analysis.)[20] In 'Socialism and War', published two years earlier, Lenin had unveiled what was to be a leading Soviet doctrine in the decades ahead: that, given the nature of exploitative Western imperialism, any struggle by a colony or backward nation against its exploiters would be a just war.[21] Under such circumstances, domestic and foreign, he asked, how could an anti-militarist and pacifist policy be Marxist?

When war came to Europe in 1914, Lenin's Bolshevik wing of the Russian Social-Democratic Party took the lead of the European socialist parties and factions opposing any proletarian participation. Lenin urged the workers to transform the world war into a world revolution. In a series of tracts, Lenin stressed the differences between a properly Marxist view of war and that of the liberal bourgeoisie. In a pamphlet on 'The Disarmament Slogan', Lenin denounced the 'Kautskyite' position in favour of a post-war disarmament as 'the most vulgar opportunism', as well as bourgeois pacifism. In the generation before 1914, the European socialist parties, under the leadership of the German and French Marxists, had underlined their commitment to national defence by a citizens' militia, based on conscription and universal military training, in opposition to the professional armies of the dynastic states. In his 'Military Programme of the Proletarian Revolution', Lenin opposed the conventional militia, so long and passionately advocated by Marxists, as a bourgeois institution, while urging the formation of a proletarian militia. This became the Bolshevik program after the March revolution, and its implementation by the Kerensky government helped to bring about the Red October. Lenin also clearly foresaw the continuing necessity of a sizeable army for purely domestic purposes so long as the revolution had not passed beyond the stage of the proletarian dictatorship. Indeed, Lenin went well beyond what might be regarded as merely a prudential position: True Marxism—the Soviets would soon call this 'true Marxism', Marxism-Leninism—he declared, was based on violence, a dictatorship of the proletariat maintained by armed troops.[22] An armed proletariat would be required to make the revolution; a considerable army would be necessary, for domestic purposes, if the revolution, once successful, were to be maintained. On these scores as well, a Marxist could not be a pacifist.

There was yet another reason for such a view. From the very beginning of the Bolshevik Revolution, the question arose as to the role Soviet armed forces might play in bringing about the world communist revolution. The Bolshevik left-wing, critical of what it saw as the opportunism of the Soviet government, urged the immediate proclamation and organization of a world revolution. In a series of articles, entitled '"Left-Wing" Childishness and the Petty-Bourgeois Mentality', Lenin denounced this left-opposition, not arguing that objective conditions in the West were not sufficiently mature to produce revolution (as a pre-War orthodox Marxist would have done), but simply that until the Soviet state was much stronger, and the imperialist powers much weaker, the Red Army had to avoid war. For when Lenin determined to seize control of an overwhelmingly peasant Russia in the name of a dictatorship of the proletariat, he in fact had adopted the romantic praxis of the 1840s, while ostensibly maintaining the more prosaic orthodox theory that looked to the growing revolutionary consciousness of an increasingly impoverished proletariat for the triumph of communism. Only 'muddleheads', he suggested, failed to realize that formulas changed with conditions.[23]

Trotsky, in December 1921, reverting to the posture of his Menshevik, orthodox past, argued that outside military intervention might indeed ease a proletarian victory in Western Europe, but this could not occur until 'the revolution is mature' with respect not only to 'social relations' but also to 'political consciousness'. 'Military intervention may be likened to the forceps of an obstetrician', he observed, 'which if applied in time can reduce the birth pangs, but if brought into play prematurely can only produce a miscarriage'. Yet Trotsky had been won over to the Bolshevik praxis. While denouncing the 'impatient strategists' who wished the Red Army to bear the immense burden of the 'final and decisive conflict', arguing that Russian backwardness prevented her from following the example of Revolutionary France in waging a war against bourgeois Europe, Trotsky, like Lenin, proclaimed himself 'in principle in favor of offensive revolutionary war'.[24]

In 'Socialism and War', Lenin had quoted Clausewitz, whom he described as 'one of the profoundest writers on the problem of war', that 'war is the continuation of politics by other means', introducing a parenthetic 'i.e., violent' to describe 'other'. (Soviet and Chinese military writings frequently quote this statement, sometimes attributing it to Lenin rather than to Clausewitz, and at times giving a profound significance to Lenin's parenthetical addition.)[25] Such a view of war was a necessary companion to the neo-Marxist vision of capitalist development. Since the bourgeoisie was ever the enemy, and capitalism in its final stage inevitably meant war, Marxism-Leninism needed always to be prepared to move the revolution from the political stage of class struggle within a nation, to that of war between socialist and capitalist nations—as we shall see later in this essay.

Despite an essential agreement on the relationship between capitalism and war, controversies have persisted among Marxists on matters of military practice, on strategy and tactics. From the earliest days of the movement, as we have observed, European socialists debated as to the proper (from a Marxist standpoint) military method to be employed in achieving power for the proletariat. Some of these debates reveal, on still another front, that we are dealing with an intellectual system which—without wishing either to flatter or to patronize—can only be compared with the theologies of the great religions. It is evident that its adherents were, and are, serious-minded in accepting the precepts of a system which they believe contains the key to ultimate, universal truth. Certainly, there are hypocrites among Marxists as among the followers of all religious and quasi-religious systems; but, as we shall see, there have always been serious efforts to define and to justify practice in terms of theory. Of course, Marxist leaders, like those who preside over other religious and ideological movements, permit pragmatic considerations to triumph over doctrinal principle, particularly where questions of power are at issue.

The critical question of how power was to be achieved presented itself in two forms. The first concerned the proletarian revolution that was to develop in the cities of Europe, and centred on the question of the effectiveness of what might be called a barricades strategy. The second did not originally concern a proletarian revolution, but a popular, predominantly rural, uprising, against a foreign invader: the issue here was whether a guerrilla strategy mounted by natives in backward regions could defeat a disciplined European army. In the former case, the one most characteristic of nineteenth century discussion, the enemy was capitalism; in the latter, predominantly but not exclusively in twentieth-century debate, it was imperialism. In the early years of our century, in Russia, the tactical questions of urban insurrection and guerrilla warfare were merged into one—as a seeming prelude to the special place that irregular war was to have in the communist strategy of our times.

The Tactics of Revolution: Barricades and Guerrilla Warfare

In the early months of 1848, a new technique of insurrection was employed in the capital cities of Europe. Barricades—fortifications made of stones from roadways, timber, etc.—were erected on the main streets. The regular armies of Europe were at first unable to counter this tactic of the rebels, artisans, and workmen, who fought behind these fortifications with such determination. The appropriate military reply to urban barricades was at last worked out by the French General Cavaignac in June 1848, and the grave threat they had once posed to the established order, although revived now and again in rhetorical flourishes, gradually evaporated.[26] For all practical purposes, the Social-Democratic Parties of Europe before 1914 sought victory in exploiting the increasing pauperization of the masses, which they were convinced would grow out of the mounting economic contradictions of capitalism. By 1894, shortly before his death, Engels was to dismiss completely the romantic yearnings for a revival of the barricades strategy of 1848—however useful such tactics might be in stimulating morale and even in winning the soldiers over to the revolution—as bound to fail when opposed by well-trained troops. If the bourgeoisie could not prevent an inevitable proletarian victory by military means (which was a conclusion of the *Anti-Dühring*), neither could the proletariat achieve it by violence. At this time, Engels urged the superiority of political weapons such as universal suffrage to accomplish proletarian objectives.[27]

Engels and Marx also wrote, and at some length, about guerrilla warfare, at first in connection with its employment against Napoleon's troops in Spain and in Russia, and then with its usefulness in Asia and Africa against Western colonial armies. Their conclusions as to the effectiveness of such a strategy were mixed. In 1857, in a discussion of the British wars in China and Persia, Engels suggested that these countries would not be successful in their efforts to import Western military techniques; only by guerrilla tactics, he declared, might they succeed in driving the British from Asia. Again, during the final months of the Indian Mutiny in 1858, Marx and Engels were critical of a British strategy that seemed bound to spur a troublesome and possibly fatal guerrilla warfare; as it happened, this never developed. Yet when Engels wrote of the Moorish War against Spain in 1860, a war in which the Moorish tribesmen did in fact employ a guerrilla strategy, Engels could only ascribe Spain's difficulties to lack of resolution on the part of the Spanish Marshal, O'Donnell. For a Westerner convinced of the progressive nature of historical development, perhaps particularly for a German, well-disciplined European regulars, bearing the marks of a superior civilization and an advanced military science, ought always to triumph over irregular 'semi-savages'. Still, even here, Engels concluded, more ambiguously, the best-led and most disciplined European regulars might be overcome, though not defeated in battle, by the wear and tear of guerrilla warfare—and 'the impossibility of conquering anything but the towns'. In an article concerning the break-up of the French regulars into guerrilla contingents after the early Prussian victories in 1870, Engels was even to write of this development as belonging to a new era of people's wars inaugurated by the American Revolution.[28]

At the beginning of the twentieth century, however, it was none the less taken for granted in Marxist circles that neither such sporadic armed uprisings nor barricade fighting would play a decisive role in the proletarian revolution, and that all kinds of irregular warfare could easily be put down by a professional army. Moreover, both barricade and guerrilla tactics appeared akin to the program of assassinations, robberies, and dynamitings, advocated by anarchists or, in Russia, by populist terrorists like Nechaev and his followers. Orthodox Marxism pronounced itself against such criminal activities, which seemed to rely on individual daring rather than broad, historically determined movements of the masses. Nevertheless, in 1905, in reaction to the defeats of Tsarist forces in the war with Japan, general strikes broke out in a number of Russian cities; barricades were raised in the classical fashion, and the populace fought a disheartened soldiery. The strikers were surprisingly successful, and in Moscow, a comparatively few men behind street fortifications managed to immobilize an entire army.

The leader of the Bolshevik faction of the Russian Social

Democratic Party, Lenin, hailed the 'new barricade tactics', which he saw as those of guerrilla warfare supplemented by 'mass terror'. Karl Kautsky, the German Social-Democratic leader, heir to Engels's authority within German Marxism, and up to then an adherent of the position that the ballot not the bomb would prove the decisive weapon, now saw the possibility that such tactics might prove successful in Western Europe as well.[29] Thus we see that in the period when military means did not seem to be a *technically* feasible method of gaining power, Marxists had declared their reliance on historical development; on the other hand, when the 1905 uprisings provided the hope for a more rapid triumph, European Marxists were not slow to accept a posture with which they had up to then been in ideological opposition. But, of course, in this they were merely following the pragmatic example of Engels whose 1848 faith in a barricades strategy had been spoiled by Cavaignac.

Still, Lenin, not unlike other Marxist leaders, continued to distrust irregular activities. Some fifteen years later, during a Civil War in which guerrilla actions were on occasion the only possible ones, Lenin none the less declared that 'the guerrilla spirit, its vestiges, remnants and survival' were the cause of 'misfortune, disintegration, defeats, [and] disasters'.[30] Yet, like Kautsky in 1906, he had been ready to accept the possible usefulness of such tactics provided that—and in this qualification we see a leading reason for Lenin's distaste—the party could place them 'under its control'. In military as in political tactics, Lenin was, and continued to be, a pragmatist. He denounced the Marxist 'systematizers' who 'in the seclusion of their studies' attempted to impose upon the masses a particular form of revolutionary warfare. Marxist military tactics, Lenin argued, would be formulated not by theoreticians and 'systematizers' but by observing 'mass practice'—the tactics spontaneously developed by the people, as in 1905. 'To attempt to answer yes or no to the question whether any particular means of struggle should be used, without making a detailed examination of the given movement at the given stage of its development, means completely to abandon the Marxist position', he declared.[31]

So we see that, in the years before 1914, Lenin had defended guerrilla tactics against the rigid orthodoxy of the Marxist 'systematizers' who had denounced them. During the years of Civil War which followed the Bolshevik Revolution of 1917, the Russian 'systematizers' were completely to reverse their earlier position. If previously a guerrilla strategy had been declared un-Marxist, a new generation of Marxist 'systematizers' now wished to translate the Bolshevik view of revolutionary theory and practice into military doctrine, and proclaimed that *only* a guerrilla strategy was appropriate to the proletariat in its effort to achieve power. The chief spokesman for a pragmatic military policy during this period was the Minister of War, Leon Trotsky. Despite Lenin's support, Trotsky was hard pressed by an opposition that included a number of the outstanding military figures of the time, including Michael Frunze and the future Marshal Tukhachevsky, who were said to have enjoyed the covert support of Stalin. The new 'systematizers', for whom the waging of war was a science to which Marxism possessed the key, saw the issue as one between their genuinely proletarian military doctrine, and the haphazard, suspiciously bourgeois strategy followed by Trotsky. They particularly denounced the tactics of positionalism, epitomized by the rigid lines on the Western front in 1914–18, in favour of the so-called 'Marxist tactics' of manœuvre. (Proponents of mechanized warfare, military theorists like J. F. C. Fuller and Liddell Hart, were soon also to extol the tactics of manœuvre as a counter to the indecisiveness of modern trench warfare.) They wished, in addition, to replace the effete bourgeois strategy of defence by one of attack, holding it to be un-Marxist even to attempt to construct or to defend fortified positions.

Trotsky excoriated this effort to endow military doctrine with a 'metaphysical spirit', accepting more or less the approach of the early Engels. The Red Army had, indeed, adopted a strategy of manœuvre, he asserted, not on doctrinal grounds, but only because of its own backwardness and that of Russian society generally, and because of the nature of the Civil War. The strategy of 'attack' was not proletarian but that of Marshal Foch and the French general staff, Trotsky insisted, while making a neat comparison which exposed the virtual identity of Frunze's so-called 'proletarian' tactics and those of the great eighteenth-century Tsarist general Suvarov—just as Engels had understood the identity of the tactics of the Theban Epaminondas and Frederick the Great. Marxism could instruct its followers when to fight, not how to fight, he continued. 'There is not and there never has been a military "science"'. On military questions, there was no 'absolute solution', merely 'empirical generalizations', and he asserted further that 'only hopeless doctrinaires believe that answers to questions of mobilization, formation, training, education, strategy and tactics can be obtained deductively, in a formal logical manner from the premises of a sacred "military doctrine"'. Military strategy and tactics were to be formulated, Trotsky argued, on the basis of military experience, not Marxist method. They were to be derived not from 'a proletarian world-outlook but from the condition of technology.' While the Red Army might be compelled to follow a strategy of 'manœuvre' when it was weak, it could and should advance to one of 'position' when it grew stronger. Trotsky pointed out that the Red Army had learned this manœuvrist strategy from the cavalry tactics of the Whites who had adopted it because they had greater skill and fewer numbers than the Reds. To suggest that a strategy of position was un-Marxist, Trotsky warned, might well undermine proletarian revolutions in advanced Western countries where 'positionalism will occupy a far more prominent place than in our civil war.' To further horrify the opposition, Trotsky declared that what the Soviets required was not a unified, proletarian military doctrine, but good platoon officers.[32]

The extended and often bitter controversy between Trotsky and the left-wing opposition had a somewhat unreal quality, for the systematizers of the left-opposition seemed less concerned with changing the actual strategy adopted by Trotsky and Lenin, than they were with pressing the need to formulate a 'unified military doctrine' of a Marxist and proletarian character. Were Frunze and Tukhachevsky, regarding themselves as more rigorous Bolsheviks than Trotsky, a recent convert from Menshevism, attempting to undermine his position as Minister of War? Were they expressing dissatisfaction with Trotsky's clearly unproletarian policy (which, incidentally, Lenin supported, accusing its opponents of 'left-wing infantilism') of employing former Tsarist officers in the Red Army, a policy in good part responsible for the Soviet victory over the Whites? Perhaps. We cannot, however, dismiss as a motive the profound discomfort experienced by true believers of an all-encompassing philosophy, that at a time when proletarian theories of painting, poetry, or engineering, physics, biology, etc. were being developed by the practitioners of those arts and sciences, the Civil War was being prosecuted without benefit of a 'proletarian' military science. Trotsky repeatedly urged the opposition to describe their military programme, but the systematizers had little to offer beyond vague generalizations advocating manœuvre over positionalism. What they found intolerable, one might speculate, was the apparent heresy of Trotsky's insistence that Marxist philosophy had nothing to say on what was, after all, a leading concern of the period between 1917 and 1922. The opposition might have been somewhat mollified if the War Minister had but given lip-service to the need to formulate such a doctrine, instead of lecturing them on the foolishness of trying to do so.

In 1924, Trotsky reviewed a newly published collection of articles on the Franco-Prussian War that Engels had written in 1870–1. Trotsky regretted that this collection, which had appeared the previous year, had not been available earlier, at a time when it might have proved useful in his struggle with the systematizers. For it was clear from these articles, Trotsky observed, that Engels had entirely shared his empirical posture; indeed, the German Marxist had even stressed the prime importance of good platoon officers![33] It is very doubtful, however, that Trotsky's opposition would have been cowed by these 1870 writings. This is apparent from the revival of the controversy, under somewhat altered circumstances, in China in the 1920s and 1930s. Although the precise terms of the argument were distributed in a different manner, the underlying issue—whether there existed a Marxist 'science' of war—was much the same.

The 'military science' of these Chinese Marxist systematizers (of men like Li Li-san and Wang Ming) received the support of Stalin, now the dominant figure in the Soviet regime, who had supposedly also been sympathetic to Frunze and his associates. Their doctrine had been derived in part from their analysis of the grounds for Soviet successes in the war against the White Army, and in part from their interpretation of the old orthodoxies of both Engels and Kautsky. These early formulators of the 'Marxist' strategy of the Chinese Communist party proclaimed the primary importance of capturing the cities—a combination of a Putschist and barricades strategy—where were to be found all that there was of the Chinese proletariat, before extending communist rule to the countryside. This was of course the way events had, more or less, unfolded in Russia. In the tradition of the orthodox Marxism of Europe, moreover, they denounced the anarchist tactics of guerrilla warfare, as being of peasant origin. Such tactics, they pointed out, had long been pursued in China by petty war lords and bandit chieftains, and were therefore particularly abhorrent in a proletarian revolution. In line with such views, Li Li-san and his comrades, during the period when they controlled the Chinese Communist Party, defended the strategy of 'positionalism', unlike Frunze and the Soviet systematizers, and wished to bring ever greater amounts of territory under the control of the Red Army, rather than accept a 'manœuvrist' strategy in which the capture of territory was of little importance. They straddled the two camps by asserting a strategy of proletarian 'attack', as had Frunze, while condemning the 'manœuvrist' avoidance of battle even when outnumbered. Of course, the Li Li-san group had misread both Lenin and Trotsky's thoroughly pragmatic management of the war, and the replies of the Bolshevik leaders to the left-systematizers, for a military orthodoxy.

The Chinese 'opposition' to what was for some years the official military policy of the party hierarchy was headed by Mao Tse-tung. At first, Mao defended, as had Lenin and Trotsky, a commonsense, pragmatic doctrine. Arguing on the basis of China's quasi-feudal, semi-colonial conditions, he espoused a guerrilla policy which sought battle only when the Red Army was superior to an enemy force, and which preferred to maintain its numbers in the relative security of the countryside rather than to court defeat in the cities, where the enemy could most easily bring superior strength to bear. Such a strategy and such tactics were appropriate to the circumstances in which China found itself, Mao argued. When the relative strength of the Red Army increased—that is, when the enemy's forces had been worn away by 'protracted war'—guerrilla tactics would be abandoned in favour of a more orthodox, positionalist strategy. In all this Mao, whether consciously or not, was recapitulating Trotsky's analysis. Mao soon found himself at the head of the party and the army, and his pragmatic strategy proved successful. The Red Armies helped to defeat the Japanese invaders, and then overcame the war-weary Nationalist forces of Chiang Kai-shek.

During the course of these wars, Mao elaborated the theory of his manœuvrist, guerrilla tactics and strategy in a series of well-written and well-argued tracts. Those works have served as the military handbooks for guerrilla movements throughout the Third World in the decades after 1945. Mao did not originate these tactics. Indeed, they had a long history, as we have already noted. Insofar as they had a Chinese flavour, this could be accounted for by the influence of Sun Tsu, a Chinese military theorist of the third century BC, whom Mao had read and admired. They were certainly in no way deduced from Marxist theory. Yet, because of their success in China, their identification with Mao as his chief contribution to theory (to be a theorist was a useful attribute for a would-be member of a pantheon that included Marx and Lenin) as well as the evident usefulness of such tactics in the formerly colonial world, they were to acquire—in China particularly, but elsewhere as well—a special aura as the method by which communist revolutions might be achieved.[34] What had begun as a pragmatic response to the Marxist systematizers became in effect a new 'system'.

Unlike the Soviet Union, Communist China had relatively small hopes of gaining control over the Communist parties of Europe, but in the undeveloped rural countries of Asia, Africa, and Latin America, a guerrilla strategy would be more useable and China's political authority more readily exerted. It was Lin Piao, Mao's old comrade-in-arms and, at the time of Lin's death in 1971, his designated successor, who proclaimed, with Mao's approval, the strategy and tactics which had brought about the capture of power in China as *the* Marxist military science. For Lin, Engels's prediction in the *Anti-Dühring*, that the 'emancipation of the proletariat' would find 'its specific expression in military affairs and create its specific, new military method' had at last been realized. More significantly, Lin also made a transformation of military into political science. Basing his analysis neither on political or economic conditions nor on the dialectical materialist view of the historical process, but rather on the 'whole range of strategy and tactics of people's war' begot by the Chinese Revolution, with its supposed roots in Marxist-Leninist theory, Lin created a new vision of Marxism-Leninism. Since the proletariat had failed to deliver the cities to communism in China—as envisaged in the Li Li-san line—Marxist-Leninists must no longer make the working-class the focus of their strategy of power. Nor had the proletariat been more forthcoming elsewhere in the Third World, or, for that matter, in the West. The new focus of historical concern was to be the peasantry. Cities throughout the world were the abode of the enemy; they were certainly where the enemy was strongest and could bring his greatest force to bear. The Maoist strategy of the 1930s had stressed the critical importance of the peasantry, and of the establishment of rural-base areas. 'To rely on the peasants, build rural base areas, and use the countryside to encircle and finally capture the cities—such was the way to victory in the Chinese revolution', Lin proclaimed. The final victory of communism over bourgeois capitalism and imperialism throughout the world would be achieved by applying these tactics on a global scale. Lin called upon the peasantry, upon the rural areas of the world (Asia, Africa, and Latin America) to rise up against 'the cities of the world' (North America and Western Europe), urging them to employ a guerrilla strategy to encircle these 'cities' and to conquer them.[35]

Trotsky had warned the left-systematizers in Russia that their strictures against a strategy of positionalism as un-Marxist might well result in the undermining of proletarian chances for victory in the West, where a positionalist strategy might prove much more feasible than in Civil War Russia. Little could he have imagined that a successful guerrilla strategy in Asia would dispossess the proletariat from its appointed role in bringing about a communist victory—at least in the programme of the Marxist–Leninist party presiding over the most populous of the earth's nations. The leadership of the Communist party in Cuba, in control of a nation with one of the smallest populations, was prepared to go even further in subordinating the orthodox political and economic analyses of Marxism to a military one, creating what may be described as a Cromwellian model of Marxism–Leninism. Régis Debray, a young Frenchman who had studied in Paris with the Marxist philosopher, Louis Althusser, taught philosophy in Havana after Castro's coming to power, and took upon himself the task of systematizing the military strategy which had brought about a communist victory in Cuba. Debray, who was to join Che Guevara in his guerrilla war against Bolivia in the mid-sixties, was in agreement with much of what Lin had said. For Debray, as well, a guerrilla strategy was the Marxist science of revolution in the twentieth century. He, too, saw the revolution as necessarily beginning in the countryside and then extending to the less congenial cities. The Cuban Marxists, Debray argued, had developed a military strategy which conformed to Marxist–Leninist doctrine and was more suitable for successful action (outside the industrialized West) than that drawn from either the Soviet or the Maoist models.

While advocating a guerrilla strategy, Debray dismissed what he described as the theory of 'armed self-defense', a spontaneous effort of a population to resist its oppressors. Only the Trotskyites—whose military views in the Latin America of the 1950s and 1960s must be distinguished from those of Trotsky himself—obsessed with 'a medieval metaphysic' (which was Debray's description of orthodox, pre-1914 Marxism!), persisted in the futile strategy of self-defence. Such a set of tactics he compared to the outworn political notion of a mass party, and just as Lenin had abandoned such an instrument in favor of a trained élite of dedicated militants, so Debray (following the example of Castro and Guevara) advocated 'the armed unit, which was organically separate from the civilian population . . . a popular regular army with its own mobility and initiative'. The Cubans had rejected the Maoists' idea of establishing a guerrilla base, the French philosopher observed. Such a base was merely an invitation for attack; the guerrilla 'armed unit' must choose 'extreme mobility'. This opting for a strategy of manœuvre, Debray continued, did not mean that one of position ought not to be adopted in the later phases of the struggle. In this, he was in agreement with Trotsky and Mao.

Debray's depiction of what he regarded as the Cuban Revolution's most valuable contribution to Marxist-Leninist military and political doctrine would have horrified Marx and Lenin, Stalin and Mao. In the view of the Cuban Marxists, the guerrilla force was not to be subordinated to the urban political leadership: neither the middle-aged Marxist theorist nor the party functionary, but the young militants of the army, 'proletarianized' by their experiences in the mountains, whatever their class background and however ignorant of revolutionary theory they might be, constituted the vanguard of the revolution. (This Cuban view was exported to Marxist guerrilla movements in South America in the sixties; in the seventies, it was welcomed, along with Cuban 'volunteers,' by the 'Marxist' military leaders of Africa.) 'Eventually the future people's Army will beget the party of which it is to be, theoretically the instrument: essentially the party is the army', Debray proclaimed. And, giving primacy to the begetter, the army was the party. Nor was the army to be managed by the Leninist principle of democratic centralism, but by its disciplined obedience to its Commander. Thus, finally, there would end '"a divorce of several decades" duration between Marxist theory and revolutionary practice', Debray continued. (The scientific theory of 'the Economist' was to be overpowered by the revolutionary heroism of 'the General'.) This 'union of theory and practice', Debray observed, was 'not an inevitability but a battle'; it must be brought about by a guerrilla movement, for 'if this union is not achieved there, it will not be achieved anywhere.'[36]

Lenin had warned that a guerrilla movement that was outside the control of the party would produce terrorism and anarchy —and, inescapably, defeat for its revolutionary purpose. The Cubans, whose spokesman Debray was, were advocates not of guerrilla anarchy—which is, no doubt, what they regarded as the consequence of 'armed self-defence'—but of what can only be called the revolutionary, military model established by

Oliver Cromwell during the English Civil Wars of the seventeenth century. Marxist theorists, and, after successful revolutions, Marxist politicians had always feared the emergence of a Cromwell or a Napoleon from the ranks of the military, ready to snatch away the fruits of proletarian success. The Cuban Marxist revolutionary tactics—in a marvellous synthesis of the military and political arms, whose collaboration had always been marked by prickly uncertainties—saw such a union of the two that the political leadership not only of the revolution, but of the future communist state, would be the product (almost by the processes of Darwinian natural selection) of the rigours of the years of guerrilla struggle. The Cromwell (or Castro) of the Revolution would rightfully exercise the political control secured by his own military successes, because these latter had most suitably prepared him to preside over a communist state.

After Castro's victory, the Cuban socialists, out of necessity (economic, political, and military) became loyal supporters and allies of Soviet Russia. But this does not appear to have affected the Russian view of their military strategy. On the whole, the Russians preferred to sanctify Michael Frunze as the great Soviet military theorist, rather than to enshrine his strategy of manœuvrism as Marxist military science. Indeed, possibly because of their hostility towards Mao's China, Soviet military theorists in recent years have tended to deal somewhat summarily with guerrilla tactics—with what the Maoists have called 'people's war'—even when discussing movements of national liberation in the formerly colonial world. Lin Piao suggested in his tract that this was because the Soviet Union had 'no faith in the masses'.

Lin also denounced those whom he called 'the Khrushchev revisionists' for their cautious view of nuclear war. 'The Marxist-Leninists and revolutionary people never take a gloomy view of war,' Lin added, concluding that 'war can temper the people and push history forward'; 'in this sense, war is a great school.'[37] After the deposition of Khrushchev in 1964, Soviet military theorists, as we shall see, threw overboard many of the more 'gloomy'—and cautious—doctrines with which they had been briefly flirting and returned to what must be regarded as the central Marxist-Leninist faith on the subject of war. Very much in the spirit of Lin and Debray, they appeared to see the school of war as the means by which the working classes of the West might be proletarianized, and a final victory over an exploitative capitalism and imperialism finally achieved.

Soviet Marxism and a Nuclear Strategy

We have discussed the effort in the Russian and Chinese Civil Wars, and subsequently, to construct a unified military doctrine. This had the look of a serious movement, but after the silencing of the opposition to Joseph Stalin's personal rule, comparatively little was heard of it. Stalin was cast in the mould of Serge Eisenstein's depiction, in his 1938 film, of the thirteenth-century feudal prince, Alexander Nevsky, who led the men of Novgorod against the Teutonic Knights, meanwhile keeping the Tartar hordes in the East at bay, to be dealt with after the defeat of the Germans. Like Eisenstein's Nevsky, Stalin was depicted as the national hero, and later the generalissimo in the 'Great Patriotic War', the descendant not only of the medieval prince of Novgorod but of the subject of another Eisenstein film, *Ivan the Terrible*. There had been faint echoes of the Frunze posture in Nevsky's announced strategy of 'rouse the peasants', and 'we must not speak of defense, but of attack', but the mood was that of Great Russian nationalism, not Marxism. During these years, military writers made relatively few efforts to produce a Marxist military science, though the enterprise was never entirely abandoned.[38]

After the explosion of the first atomic bombs, during the period when the United States and Britain possessed a monopoly of the means of nuclear warfare, Stalin fielded two contradictory policies: one suggested that atomic weapons had not genuinely altered the character of modern war—as he put it, that they could only impress people with weak nerves; another attempted to mobilize world opinion against the immoral use of so terrible a weapon. Both lines had the effect of weakening whatever leverage an atomic monopoly might give the West. At the same time, in private conversation, Stalin was reported to have spoken, in quasi-messianic terms, of a Third World War, which would be the final war between the socialist and imperialist camps, with the palms of victory inevitably falling to communism.[39] After Russia had exploded its first hydrogen bomb in 1953, the Soviets continued to play down the revolutionary character of nuclear armaments while at the same time using their possession by Russia as a threat against the West. After Stalin's death, however, there appears to have been a debate among his successors on the matter. One group, whose spokesman was Malenkov, saw the final battle between the two camps as one that might well end with the destruction of civilization rather than just of imperialism. Nikita Khrushchev, holding the same view, was to suggest in discussions with the Chinese in the late 1950s that 'the atom bomb recognizes no class distinctions.'

Krushchev, most clearly in the early sixties, had, apparently, been won over to a view of modern nuclear war that was more or less like the dominant view of American strategists of the time. He had concluded that the widespread devastation of nuclear war would prove so calamitous to both Russia and America that the West would not venture to make a surprise attack. Such an opinion did not prevent Krushchev from using the threat of atomic devastation against a West in which he believed a pacifist public opinion could be easily cowed. Like the American strategists, Khrushchev saw missiles as the basis of a Soviet defence, and, by thus substituting fire-power for manpower, he saw no necessity for the billions spent on Russia's enormous army, or the securing of a large navy or air force. While a section of the military establishment had, similarly, been won over to the necessity of a 'modern' strategy in response to the new technology, not surprisingly most of the military leaders adhered to the 'traditional' position, embodied in centuries of Tsarist policy, that insisted on the continued need of a great continental power for large forces-in-being. Such a posture was natural to generals, fearful of losing their divisions; it was also useful to bureaucrats and party officials who agreed with Lenin that the dictatorship of the proletariat could only be sustained by large armed forces, as well as to the officials with a stake in the heavy-industry sector of the economy, upon which armies and navies depended. From what little we know, there is reason to believe that Khrushchev's views on military strategy were one reason for his being removed from office in November 1964.[40]

Soon after Stalin's death, the Soviet military literature once again took up the quest for the Marxist key that would solve all military problems. Recent Russian military writings are pock-marked by references to the dicta of the formulators of Marxist–Leninism. Again and again, the same quotations are brought forward, almost as a touchstone of orthodoxy, without any apparent recognition of their frequently prosaic quality, as the capstones of paragraphs or pages with which they sometimes have only the most tenuous connection. 'Nothing so depends on economic conditions, as the army and navy', wrote Engels. 'War is a continuation of policy by other [i.e., violent] means', wrote Lenin. Inevitably, Lenin is referred to much more frequently than Engels. Most often the reference to doctrine comes in the form of attributing a concept not to an individual, but to the more generalized body of doctrine of Marxism–Leninism. Clearly many of these references have a ritualistic character, but on the whole, and particularly since the death of Stalin, even if the would-be Marxist systematizers of military doctrine display no great skill in relating ideology to practical military questions, they seem serious rather than cynical in their effort to do so.

We have some sense of this effort in articles trying to harness Marxist dialectics to military science. 'The most important condition for the proper understanding of all the processes of the world, Lenin taught,' the author of one such article, a Colonel Krupnov, wrote, quoting Lenin's phrase, 'is "the understanding of them as a unity of contradictions"'. Another writer has referred to 'the well-known law of dialectics–the transition of quantity into quality.' What these writers offered, on this foundation, was sufficiently commonplace. One hardly needed Marxist dialectics to understand that new forms of attack brought into play corresponding means of defence; or that a strategic nuclear rocket strike might be construed as a 'synthesis', combining attack and defence; or that the nuclear rocket, like the machine gun and the tank earlier, was not going to revolutionize the waging of war until armies possessed them in sufficient quantities.[41] But to accept that Soviet strategists frequently reason in this fashion makes it possible to understand what might otherwise be puzzling. (For example, a recent Pentagon analysis of Soviet aircraft noted with surprise that Russia seemed to have adopted a 'mirror-image concept' in their armaments programme, that is, the building of specific weapons systems to counter similar systems in the American inventory; this has been the kind of response that the US defence establishment, primarily concerned with creating entirely new types of aircraft, has sought to avoid.[42] But Soviet strategists have explicitly urged the mounting of such counters—contradictions or antitheses—as precisely what Marxist dialectics required. No doubt, such military programmes would have to be otherwise justifiable or else they would not pass muster with the professionals who we must assume know their trade; that, or risk being dismissed as having been improperly arrived at—the work of amateurs, mere ideologues with no genuine understanding of the military art.)

Contemporary Soviet military theorists, like Engels and Lenin, begin with Clausewitz: war is a continuation of politics by other means. They dismiss the view of many Western military theorists that, because of the destructive character of nuclear warfare, this Clausewitzian principle has been outmoded, attributing such an opinion to the 'metaphysical and anti-scientific' approach of Western thinking. For the Marxist, they argue, the essential nature of war as a continuation of politics has not altered with changing technology and armaments. They condemn what they regard as the idealization of the nuclear bomb, which they suggest has had the effect of transferring the control of war from the political leaders to the military.[43]

Given the dominant tendency of Marxist historiography, and the military doctrine of the *Anti-Dühring*, we might have expected Soviet and Chinese military writers to view war overwhelmingly in terms of technological development. But this has clearly not been the case. Perhaps the most noteworthy contemporary economic-determinist view of war is to be found in the writings of the non-Marxist British strategist, tactician, and military historian, J. F. C. Fuller. Curiously, the makers of Soviet military doctrine—who were so much influenced by Fuller's views on tank warfare in the 1920s through the 1940s—make him a particular target of attack for his elevating the importance of equipment over morale. In this, like Marx, Engels, and Lenin, they follow Clausewitz. Moreover, from the standpoint of dialectical materialism, war-time morale has been enlisted by Soviet military theorists to play the role traditional Marxist theory had assigned to the immiseration of the proletariat. What will assure a communist victory in the coming struggle, Soviet strategists argue, will be the high morale of communist societies as compared with the West. Western morale would be further depressed, they add, by a war whose strains would increasingly reveal the inadequacies of bourgeois society.[44]

Are Soviet theorists, remembering that the turmoil of the First World War had made possible that most unlikely event, given orthodox Marxist theory, a communist revolution in Russia, therefore turning almost as a last hope to a Third World War which would so shatter bourgeois society as to overcome the failure of objective economic conditions to bring about a social revolution? This at times appears to be the mood of contemporary Soviet military doctrine. One authoritative Soviet work quotes Marx as having written that 'such is the redeeming feature of war; it puts a nation to the test. As exposure to the atmosphere reduces all mummies to instant dissolution, so war passes supreme judgment upon social organizations that have outlived their vitality.' The Soviet commentator observed, in support of Marx, that the strain engendered by the 'enormous exertion of all material and spiritual forces' not only shattered Tsarist Russia in 1917, but both Germany and Italy in the Second World War. War, this military spokesman added, 'subjects to a stern test the firmness and viability of political systems. Systems that had seemed all-powerful and unshakeable often turn out to be rotten through and through'.[45] Thus, in a nuclear age, we encounter a revival of Social Darwinism, in Marxist vestments.

A twentieth-century Marxist, of course, might understand the emphasis on morale as the dialectical infiltration of the subjective element into praxis, but a less subtle interpretation may be more persuasive. For, given long-time American technological superiority, this Soviet view is as understandable as the pre-1914 French high command's glorification of attack by bayonet, in an effort to counter German superiority in both numbers and economic development. Mao Tse-tung also extolled the importance of morale, and, indeed, of the role of the individual in warfare:[46] how else could he have hoped for victory against the superior and more plentiful equipment of both the Japanese and Chiang's armies? (Under Mao, Chinese military doctrine appeared to see bayonets in the hands of an enthusiastic soldiery as capable of opposing tanks. However, a military spokesman has lately observed that while 'we stress people's war and human factors', the Chinese Red Army now saw the importance of improving 'weapons and equipment' and 'technological conditions'. Moreover, the most recent Chinese military doctrine has denounced as 'absurd' Mao's guerrilla strategy of 'luring the enemy in deep' if China were attacked.)[47] Engels himself, for similar reasons, had made a demurral on behalf of an 'idealist' morale over materialist technological factors even in his otherwise doctrinaire *Anti-Dühring*. (And Engels, we remember, had also spoken hopefully of the revolution emerging from the disorders accompanying a world war.)

The Soviets, moreover, have borrowed the distinction which late nineteenth- and early twentieth-century Italian and German anticipators of national socialism had conceived between 'capitalist' nations, like England, and 'proletarian' nations like Germany and Italy. The Soviet strategists now see class struggle as existing not only between proletarians and capitalists within the nations of the bourgeois West, but also on an international plane, between socialist and imperialist camps. They proclaim that the new technology of war has made possible the achievement of 'the most decisive political goals'. A future world war between the socialist and imperialist camps would take on the keen class ferocity of a revolutionary civil war. It would be a 'decisive armed collision of two opposing world social systems'—and here the literature frequently assumes an apocalyptic tone: the contradictions between these systems were more profound, and consequently, the wars between them would be more destructive than all previous conflicts.

Along with a conviction of the necessity of a 'class' war between the socialist and imperialist camps—for the Marxist military literature (Soviet and Maoist, in both the communist bloc and in the West) reiterates the themes set down by

Luxemburg and the neo-Marxists, by Bukharin and Lenin—we find a Marxist faith in the inevitability of a socialist victory. This faith is central to Marxism, to the dialectical interpretation of historical development. History assures the Marxist that reactionary capitalism is doomed to destruction: there will come an Armageddon—the Russian Marshal Sokolovskii prophesied that 'entire states will be wiped off the face of the earth'—a final struggle between the Children of Light and the Children of Darkness, and victory would belong to the 'progressive' forces of communism against those who battle in vain against the foreordained and inexorable path of History. This victory, moreover, would not be gained through mere technological superiority, but because the peoples of the West, finally perceiving the vicious selfishness of their ruling classes, would join the socialist camp in their just war against the forces of reaction.[48]

The Triumph of Military Science Over Marxism?

To sum up, Soviet military doctrine, for nearly two decades now, has pushed aside the doubts of those in the military who had supported Khrushchev's policy of deterrence, on the grounds that a nuclear war would destroy both the socialist and imperialist camps. Rather, they have insisted that were such a war to take place—if the West were either to attack or by its provocative behavior compel the Soviet Union to launch a defensive attack—then the socialist camp would inevitably win. They have dismissed as un-Marxist the view that the Clausewitzian dictum that war was but the continuation of politics had been invalidated by nuclear technology. War was still war. Indeed, only through war—and this seemed the implicit argument of Soviet strategists—could a lethargic working class in the West be spurred to accomplish its proletarian mission. The syllogism is clear if as yet incomplete: because of the nature of capitalism, war is inevitable; in such a war, however devastating, the socialist camp must prove victorious; the third, and concluding term of the argument cannot be reassuring, however it may be stated.

In 1961, when Khrushchev's position on deterrence still carried weight in Soviet circles, one of the more perceptive

American observers of Russia, George Kennan, wrote: 'The Marxist–Leninist ideology did not suggest that it was by a single grand military conflict between the world of Communism and the world of capitalism that these aims were to be achieved.' 'In the course of the last twenty years,' Kennan continued—describing his efforts to explain 'the Soviet threat' —'in no respect have I found it so difficult to obtain understanding as in the presentation of this one simple fact.' The Soviets had always stressed, Kennan insisted, that socialism would triumph through the operation of social forces within bourgeois countries.[49] Unfortunately, this 'one simple fact' has been cast into further doubt in the last fifteen years. Yet Kennan's primary conclusion, albeit from what now appears a dubious premise, may still be valid—that a pre-emptive war, quite apart from its frightful cost in lives, would create more problems than it would solve. Nor ought we to assume that the present Soviet view, however disturbingly well-founded in Marxist–Leninist theory, will not be altered. But the threat presented by such a position cannot be lightly disregarded.

There is, as we have seen, evidence other than the new Soviet method for proletarianizing the working class in the West to persuade us that traditional Marxism is undergoing a dangerous transformation. The Soviet revival of the revolutionary strategy of 1848, in a global form, is but one aspect of the new face of Marxism. The terrorism which has beset the West for over a decade, often implemented by men and women who think of themselves as Marxists, is perhaps the most dramatic instance of this revival, to use the terminology of the left-Hegelians of the 1840s (and of the Frankfurt School of the middle decades of our century) of the subjective, heroic component of praxis. Although Marxists still speak of the objective, economic contradictions which will rouse the proletariat to revolution, for the Soviets such contradictions will only be made apparent by war, as happened in Russia in 1914–17; for the Chinese communists, they will be made evident by a global assault of the peasantry of the countryside upon the cities, on the model of what occurred in China, in the 1930s and 1940s. The 'Marxist' terrorists, who appear to think themselves as following the teaching of the leaders of the Frankfurt school, particularly of Marcuse, by individual attacks on the weak points of the complex bourgeois societies, have revived the tactics of Bakunin, which Marx had censured, and those of the Russian populist terrorists like Nechaev, which Plekhanov and even Lenin had denounced.

Most recently, in Cuba, as we have seen, orthodox Marxist theory has been so much altered to bring it into line with military praxis that we may speak of a new 'military Marxism', one which has explicitly discarded much of the traditional theory in favour of one frankly established on a military model. Régis Debray, the chief spokesman for this new theory, has written of the victory of Cuban Marxism as signifying 'the death of a certain ideology', one characteristic of an era of 'relative class equilibrium', and the beginning of a new one of 'total class warfare'. The time for trade unions, reformism, and 'compromise solutions' had passed; history had moved to a new stage of 'struggle to the death'. The Marxism-Leninism of the Cuban Revolution had given up its hopes in a proletariat that had been bourgeoisified by the cities, and in the leaders of trade unions and Marxist parties who inevitably tended toward becoming cautious and self-protecting reformists. The traditional view, Debray declared, was 'an abstract metaphysic, a concept with no grasp of history', and was doomed to defeat. The inevitable triumph of the proletariat would be brought about by military means, rather than by those predicted by orthodox Marxism.[50]

The only viable solution for Marxists has seemed to be a turn to the kind of military action that Marx and Engels had ridiculed when they heard it expounded by their Baden comrade Willich in the public houses of London, after the defeat of their quite similar hopes by General Cavaignac. The Cuban Revolution, like the Russian and the Chinese, had proved that success *was* obtainable by such means, whereas other more traditional methods had failed. In Cuba, the 'medieval metaphysic' of Marxist orthodoxy yielded before the modern cult of force, applied not in the futile fashion of sporadic uprisings of the exploited, but, on the model of the Leninist political theory, by a military élite in command of an army whose members would be proletarianized by the school of war and whose supreme leaders (both political and military) would be selected by the test of military fitness. Khrushchev might have trembled before an awesome nuclear war, but his successors appear more likely to see military means as making possible the reaching of 'the most decisive political goals'. The class-struggle would be removed from the intra-national arena, where it had proved ineffective, and transposed to an international 'decisive armed collision of two opposing world social-systems' in a Soviet version of a Darwinian 'struggle to the death'.

One must avoid the bald presumption that what had begun as an effort to discover a Marxist science of war has ended with the science of war having replaced what was once Marxism. Marxist states are now born in military coups not social revolutions. What can we think of the Brezhnev Doctrine which threatens force to prevent the loss, for any reason, of a member of the Soviet Bloc? In 1968, Soviet armies did march to suppress the 'revisionism' of the Czech communist party and state, fearing not only the withdrawal of Czechoslovakia from the Marxist-Leninist camp, but the diffusion of such dangerous sentiments; eleven years later, they moved into Afghanistan to replace one puppet ruler with another they thought more pliant. Has Engels as 'the General' triumphed over Marx 'the Economist'?

We must remember, however, that all who call themselves Marxists are not agreed on a single political or military posture, though it is hardly surprising that some Marxists, upset by the delays in the historical inevitability that was to bring them final victory, should grasp at what seems a surer means of success, or should fortify themselves with an increasing reliance upon the romantic, the millennial and apocalyptic elements always present in their faith. Moreover, given the uses of the dialectic (in both its crude and subtle versions), it is arguable that it may have been inevitable that Marxist thought on military questions should evolve in such a direction. How long will it be before we hear a Marxist reversal of the Clausewitzian formula—and discover that politics is a continuation of war by other means? This may prove to have been the contribution of the Marxist Pol Pot regime of Cambodia, or perhaps of the Marxist terrorists who view armed violence as the only weapon which can be used against what they equate, by a linguistic legerdemain, as the latent 'violence' of Western liberal political institutions. This would be a ludicrous, but not impossible, conclusion to the long effort to create a Marxist science of war.

NOTES

1 Friedrich Engels to Karl Marx, Jan. 7 1858, in Karl Marx and Friedrich Engels, *Werke* (Berlin: Dietz Verlag, 1963), xxix: 252. Hereafter cited as *Marx-Engels Werke.*

2 On Guibert, see R. R. Palmer, 'Frederick the Great, Guibert, Bülow: From Dynastic to National War', in E. M. Earle, ed., *Makers of Modern Strategy: Military Thought from Machiavelli to Hitler* (Princeton, N.J.: Princeton University Press, 1943), pp. 63-8; on von Bülow, see R. R. Palmer, 'Frederick the Great, Guibert, Bülow,' ibid., pp. 69-74; on Jomini, see Crane Brinton, Gordon A. Craig, and Felix Gilbert, 'Jomini', ibid., pp. 77-92.

3 See, for example, Engels to Joseph Weydemeyer, April 12 1853, in *Marx-Engels Werke*, xxviii: 577.

4 Marx began to read Clausewitz in the course of writing an article for an American encyclopaedia on the Prussian General Blücher. See Marx to Engels, Oct. 31 1857, *Marx-Engels Werke*, xxix: 205; and also Marx to Engels, Jan. 11 1858, xxix: 256. For an account of Marx's and Engels's speculations on military subjects, see Sigmund Neumann, 'Engels and Marx: Military Concepts of the Social Revolutionaries', in Earle, *Makers of Modern Strategy*, pp. 155-71; and the more perceptive R. Nisbet, *The Social Philosophers* (New York: Crowell, 1973), pp. 78-89.

5 See Gustav Mayer, *Friedrich Engels: A Biography* (London, 1936), pp. 134-5 and *passim.* A recent East German work deals with Engels's military activities in the late forties: H. Helmert, *Friedrich Engels—Adjutant der Revolution, 1848-49* (Leipzig, 1973); also Engels to Weydemeyer, June 19 1851, *Marx-Engels Werke*, xxvii: 554-7.

6 For the progress of Engels's military education, see letters of Engels to Weydemeyer, Aug. 7 1851; Jan. 23 1852; and April 12 1853. *Marx-Engels Werke*, xxvii: 569-71; xxviii: 452-83; and 576-7.

7 See Engels to H. J. Lincoln (Editor of the *Daily News*), March 30 1854, *Marx-Engels Werke*, xxviii: 600-3.

8 See particularly their letters in the period of 1857-8: Engels to Marx, Sept. 21 1857; Sept. 22 1857; March 16 1858, in *Marx-Engels Werke*, xxix: 180-1, 183-7, 301. And Marx to Engels, Oct. 31 1857; Jan. 11 1858; March 15 1858; in ibid., xxix: 205, 256, 300.

9 See, for example, Gerhard Zirke, *Der General. Friedrich Engels, der erste Militär-theoretiker der Arbeiterklassen* (Leipzig, 1957); and J. L. Wallach, *Die Kriegslehre von Friedrich Engels* (Frankfurt, 1968). A recent American study is Martin Berger, *Engels, Armies, and Revolution: The Revolutionary Tactics of*

Classical Marxism (Hamden, Conn: Shoe String Press, 1977). Engels military writings have been translated and published in both Russian and German: F. Engels, *Izbrannye voennye proizvedeniia* (Moscow, 1957); and F. Engels, *Ausgewählte militärische schriften* (Berlin, 1958-64), 2 vols. Engels's *New American Cyclopaedia* articles on Army, Infantry, Attack, and Battle have been published separately: *Die Armee* (Berlin: Dietz, 1956); *Die Infantrie. Der Angriff. Die Schlacht.* (Berlin: Dietz, 1956).

10 See [F. Engels] 'Army', *New American Cyclopaedia*, eds., G. Ripley and C. A. Dana (New York, 1858-63), II, 123-40; and 'Infantry', *NAC*, pp. 512-22. The apparent greater awareness of social context in the 'Infantry' article might be linked to the conception of the infantry as the plebeian or proletarian branch of the army. The article on 'Army' had, in the accepted manner, depicted the cavalry as the aristocratic arm, and the artillerymen as originally forming 'a sort of guild'. The 'artillery was considered not as an arm but a handicraft', Engels had observed, and their officers were 'more related to master-tailors and carpenters than to gentlemen.'

Marx appears to have regarded the article 'Army' as bringing out in the clearest manner the 'connection between productive forces and social relations'. Marx to Engels, Sept. 25 1857, *Marx-Engels Werke*, xxix: 192-3.

11 Engels, 'Army', *NAC*, II, 140.

12 F. Engels, *Anti-Dühring; Herr Eugen Dühring's Revolution in Science* (Moscow, 1962), Part II, Chap. IV, pp. 229-40.

13 Engels, 'Infantry', *NAC*, pp. 513, 520.

14 Engels, *Anti-Dühring*, p. 232.

15 Ibid., p. 234.

16 F. Engels, 'The Seven Weeks War', [originally published in *Manchester Guardian*, Jan. 20 1866], in *Engels as Military Critic: Articles by Friedrich Engels reprinted from the Volunteer Journal and the Manchester Guardian of the 1860s.* Introduction by W. H. Chalmer and W. O. Henderson (Manchester: Manchester University Press, 1959), p. 125; and pp. 136, 139-40. [Originally in *Manchester Guardian*, July 3 and July 6, 1866.]

17 Engels, *Anti-Dühring*, pp. 239-40.

18 Rosa Luxemburg, 'Militarism as a Province of Accumulation', *The Accumulation of Capital* (New Haven: Yale University Press, 1951), pp. 454-67. [Originally published in 1913.]

19 R. Hilferding, *Das Finanzkapital; eine studie über die jüngste Entwicklung des Kapitalismus* (Berlin: Dietz, 1955), *passim.* A summary of the argument appears on pp. 552-62. [Originally published in 1910.] Also N. Bukharin, *Imperialism and World Economy* (New York: Monthly Review Press, 1973), pp. 123-7; 139-40; and V. I. Lenin, 'Preface', ibid., p. 12. [Originally published in 1915.]

20 V. I. Lenin, *Imperialism: The Highest Stage of Capitalism* (New York: International Publishers, 1939), pp. 62-3, 82-5, 88f., 96-8, and *passim.* [Originally published in 1917.] See also P. A. Baran and P. M. Sweezy, *Monopoly Capital* (New York: Monthly Review, 1968), pp. 4-7 and *passim*; and E. Mandel, *Marxist Economic Theory* (London: Merlin Press, 1968),] pp. 441-81, 521-7, and *passim.*

21 V. I. Lenin, 'Socialism and War' (1915), *Collected Works* (Moscow: Progress Publishers, 1964-5), XXI, 301-4.

22 V. I. Lenin, 'The Disarmament Slogan', (1916), *Collected Works*, XXIII, 95; and 'The Military Program of the Proletarian Revolution' (1916), ibid., pp. 77-86.

23 V. I. Lenin, '"Left-Wing" Childishness and the Petty-Bourgeois Mentality' (1920), *Collected Works,* XXVII, 327, and *passim.*

24 L. Trotsky, 'Military Doctrine or Pseudo-Military Doctrinairism' (Dec. 5 1921), *Military Writings* (New York: Merit Publishers, 1969), pp. 51-3 and *passim.*

25 V. I. Lenin, 'Socialism and War', *Collected Works*, XXI, 304-5; see also B. Byely, G. Fyodorov, and V. Kulakov, *Marxism-Leninism on War and Army* (Moscow: Progress Publishers, 1972), pp. 16-19, 35 f., 44 ff., and *passim*. For the attribution of the slogan to Lenin, see *Selected Military Writings of Mao Tse-tung* (Peking: Foreign Languages Press, 1967), p. 266, footnote to p. 227. For Lenin's (and Stalin's) considerable debt to Clausewitz, see H. A. Kissinger, *Nuclear Weapons and Foreign Policy* (New York: Council on Foreign Relations and Harper, 1957), pp. 340-3.

26 Neumann, 'Engels and Marx', in Earle, *Makers of Modern Strategy*, pp. 159 f., and *passim*.

27 F. Engels, 'Introduction' (1895), to K. Marx, *The Class Struggles in France, 1848-50* (New York: International Publishers, 1964), pp. 21-5.

28 On Spain, see K. Marx and F. Engels, *Revolution in Spain* (New York: International Publishers, 1939), pp. 51-5. [Originally published in *New York Daily Tribune*, Oct. 30 1854.] For possible guerrilla war in Asia, see F. Engels, 'On Persia and China', in K. Marx and F. Engels, *On Colonialism* (Moscow: Foreign Languages Publishing House, n.d.), pp. 123-7. [Originally published in *New York Daily Tribune*, May 22, 1857.] On Indian mutiny: K. Marx (and F. Engels), Articles for the *New York Daily Tribune*, May 25 1858; June 15 1858; July 21 1858; Oct. 1 1858. [Written by Engels but appearing under Marx's name.] Reprinted in S. Avineri, ed., *Karl Marx on Colonialism and Modernization* (New York: Doubleday, 1968), pp. 286, 299-300; 308-9; 328-9. On Morocco, see K. Marx (and F. Engels), Articles for *New York Daily Tribune*, Jan. 19 1860; Feb. 8 1860; March 17 1860. Ibid., pp. 377-9; 383-4; 394-7. On the Franco-Prussian War, see F. Engels, 'On Guerrilla War', in W. J. Pomeroy, ed., *Guerrilla Warfare and Marxism* (New York: International Publishers, 1968), pp. 57-60 [Originally published in *Pall Mall Gazette*, Nov. 11 1870.]

29 V. I. Lenin, in *Selected Works* (New York: International Publishers, 1967), I, pp. 577-83. [Originally published in *Proletary*, Aug. 29 1906.]

30 V. I. Lenin, 'All Out for the Fight against Denikin', *Collected Works*, XXIX, p. 448.

31 V. I. Lenin, 'On Guerrilla Warfare', *Collected Works*, XI, pp. 218 f., 213 f.

32 L. Trotsky, 'Unified Military Doctrine' (Nov. 1 1921), *Military Writings*, pp. 19 f., 22-8, and *passim*; 'Military Doctrine or Pseudo Military Doctrinairism' (Dec. 5 1921), ibid., pp. 32-8, 42 f., 57, 66 f., and *passim;* 'Our Current Basic Military Tasks' (April 1 1922), ibid., pp. 72-5, 79-85, 88-91, 99-101, 103-5, and *passim*; 'Marxism and Military Knowledge' (May 8 1922), ibid., pp. 110-13; 116-21, 124-32, and *passim*. For an interesting treatment of the military disputes during the Civil War period, see E. M. Earle, 'Lenin, Trotsky, Stalin: Soviet Concepts of War', in Earle, ed., *Makers of Modern Strategy*, pp. 322-45.

33 L. Trotsky, 'Marxism and Military Warfare' (March 19 1924), ibid., pp. 134-47.

34 Mao, 'Problems of Strategy in China's Revolutionary War' (Dec. 1936) in *Military Writings*, pp. 80 f., 92 ff., 101 ff., 105 f., 111 ff., 119-21, 136-47, and *passim*; 'Problems of Strategy in Guerrilla War Against Japan' (May, 1938), ibid., pp. 167 f., 179, and *passim*; 'On Protracted War' (May, 1938), ibid., pp. 217 f., 222 ff., 225-7, 230 f., 238 f., 254 f., and *passim*.

35 Lin Piao, 'Long Live the Victory of People's War', in Jay Mallin, ed., *Strategy for Conquest* (Coral Gables, Fla.: University of Miami Press, 1970), pp. 125-8, 135-42, 146-54, 158-61, and *passim*.

36 Régis Debray, *Revolution in the Revolution?* New York: Monthly Review Press, 1967), pp. 20-5, 28-31, 36-45, 60-5, 83 f., 88-91, 95-115, 121 f. For the arrival of these ideas in Ethiopia, see *New York Times*, Dec. 4 1977, Sec. IV, p. 3.

37 Lin Piao, 'Long Live the Victory of People's War', *Strategy for Conquest*, pp. 158–61.

38 See the useful R. L. Garthoff, *How Russia Makes War: Soviet Military Doctrine* (London: Allen & Unwin, 1954), pp. 25–62, and *passim*.

39 Quoted in R. Aron, *The Imperial Republic, The United States and the World, 1945–1973* (Cambridge, Mass.: Winthrop, 1974), p. 52 f. n.

40 See H. S. Dinerstein, L. Gouré, and T. M. Wolfe, Introduction, to V. D. Sokolovskii, *Soviet Military Strategy* (Englewood Cliffs, N.J.: Rand Corp. and Prentice Hall, 1963), *passim*. Marshall Sokolovskii's book represents the victory of a 'centrist' position in the military leadership, somewhat straddling the modernists and traditionalists, but leaning toward the latter. Not only do more recent, individually signed articles in military journals confirm Sokolovskii's leading views, but so do the positions taken by the various editions of the official and jointly edited *Marxism–Leninism on War and Army*. See also *Khrushchev Remembers; The Last Testament* (Boston: Little, Brown, 1974), pp. 34–60, 220, 411, 534–7, and *passim*.

41 Col. S. I. Krupnov, 'According to the Laws of Dialectics' (from *Red Star*, Jan. 7 1966), in W. R. Kintner and H. F. Scott, *The Nuclear Revolution in Soviet Military Affairs* (Norman, Okla.: University of Oklahoma Press, 1968), pp. 235–44.

42 *New York Times*, Nov. 9 1977, p. 4.

43 See Sokolovskii, *Soviet Military Strategy*, pp. 271–4 and *passim*; and Byely, *et al.*, *Marxism–Leninism on War and Army*, pp. 16–18, 35 f., 40–57, 99–103, 193–5, 392 f., and *passim*.

44 In his writings in the 1920s, Fuller made an enormous effort to convince the British military establishment that the industrial revolution had completely altered the shape of war. Fuller, who commanded the British tank corps in the War of 1914, hoped to win over the Army (which, into the late 1920s, was spending more money for the feeding of cavalry horses than it was for petrol) to the advantages of mechanization. See V. Ye. Sovkin, *Basic Principles of Operational Art and Tactics* (US Air Force, 1972), pp. 92–7. Also see Sokolovskii, *Soviet Military Strategy*, pp. 123–30; Byely *et al.*, *Marxism–Leninism On War and Army*, pp. 57–67 and *passim*.

45 Byely *et al.*, *Marxism–Leninism on War and Army*, p. 34. Marx's statement originally appeared in a *New York Tribune* article of Sept. 24 1855.

46 Mao, *Military Writings*, pp. 225 f., and *passim*.

47 See Drew Middleton, in *New York Times*, Nov. 27 1977; also Nigel Wade, *Daily Telegraph* (London), Sept. 20 1979, p. 6.

48 See, for example, Sokolovskii, *Soviet Military Strategy*, pp. 85–140, 269–74, 309–14; Byely *et al.*, *Marxism–Leninism on War and Army*, pp. 13–15, 24–7, 48–57, 87 f., 99–103, 142, 193 ff., 392 f.

49 G. F. Kennan, *Russia and the West under Lenin and Stalin* (Boston: Little, Brown, 1961), p. 389.

50 R. Debray, *Revolution in the Revolution?*, see f.n. 36. See also two excellent recent studies by Walter Laqueur, *Guerilla* (New York, 1976) and *Terrorism* (New York, 1977).

I. MARXISM AND MILITARY ART AND SCIENCE

Friedrich Engels (1820-95), born in the Prussian city of Barmen, was the lifelong collaborator of Karl Marx, and the author, along with Marx, of the *Communist Manifesto* of 1848. Engels participated briefly in the revolutionary fighting of that year in Baden, an experience that awakened his interest in military questions in which he was to make himself a specialist. In the early 1840s, Engels had helped to manage a family-owned cotton-spinning factory near Manchester, a position to which he returned after the failure of the 1848 revolution, becoming one of the main financial supports of the Marx family after it had settled in England in 1849. Engels was also keenly interested in philosophical questions, and both his philosophical and military interests found expression in his *Herr Eugen Dühring's Revolution in Science*, which appeared in 1878.

Indeed, the classical application of Marxist principles to military affairs is to be found in the *Anti-Dühring*. In reply to Dühring's 'system', which was attracting the favorable attention of many German Socialists, Engels began a construction of a Marxist counter-system. In his 'force theory', Dühring had argued the primacy of political relations in society, with economic relationships being entirely subordinate; in insisting on the predominance of economics, Engels presented a thoroughgoing, if somewhat crudely materialist view. Armies and armaments, strategy and tactics were the products of the stage of economic development, he argued, not the '"free creations of the mind" of generals of genius'. What Engels particularly wished to demonstrate was that the economic forces that had constructed (and would soon necessarily undermine) the capitalist system could not be halted by displays of force.

Engels had been writing about military questions for nearly three decades before he had attempted this systematic view of war and militarism from the standpoint of dialectical materialism. His earlier writings give evidence of a very different, even contradictory tone. [See the introductory essay.] The reader will have the opportunity of reading some of Engels's previous writings in Section II. It is, however, this chapter of the 1878 work to which the later Marxist theorists of war, determined to construct a proletarian military science, were to refer in mounting their analyses. (Section IA.)

Leon Trotsky (1877–1940) was a Russian Social Democrat and revolutionary, and one of the chief collaborators of V. I. Lenin (see Introduction to Section III) in the making of the October Revolution of 1917. After the Bolshevik seizure of power, Trotsky became first the Foreign Minister, and in 1918 the People's Commissar for Military and Naval Affairs. During the Russian Civil War (1918–22), he organized a Red Army of nearly five million men and helped to plan its successful campaigns against the armies opposed to the Bolsheviks. After Lenin's death in 1924, Trotsky's influence declined as Stalin's rose. Stalin secured Trotsky's expulsion from Russia in 1929, and his assassination in Mexico in 1940.

During the course of the Civil War, in speeches in 1921 and 1922, Trotsky took issue with a left-group of Marxist systematizers who wished to achieve Engels's goal, as outlined in the *Anti-Dühring*, of constructing a proletarian science of war, that is, a unified Marxist military theory. (This group of Marxist synthesizers included the military theorist Michael Frunze and the future Soviet Marshal Tukhachevsky, and supposedly enjoyed the covert support of Stalin.) Trotsky denounced such an endeavour as entirely metaphysical, and urged that strategy and tactics should be based on military experience, not Marxist methodology. What the Red Army most required, Trotsky insisted, was not a unified doctrine but good platoon commanders. (Section IB, 1–3.)

The Marxist military theorists had a particular veneration for Clausewitz, particularly for his view that war was 'the continuation of politics by other means'. Carl von Clausewitz (1780–1831) was a Prussian officer who fought in his country's wars against the France of the Revolution and of Napoleon. Clausewitz was a colleague of Scharnhorst and Gneisenau in the formulating and administering of the military reforms of the first decade of the nineteenth century which prepared the Prussian army for its eventual triumph over Napoleon. (In 1812, after the invasion of Russia, he and other Prussian officers joined the Russian army to continue the war against the French Emperor.) In 1818, Clausewitz became the director of his country's war college, the Allgemeine Kriegsschule, and in the course of this service began to write on strategical questions. His most notable work, *Vom Kriege* (*On War*) was published posthumously. Marx and Engels much admired Clausewitz, whose views carried the aura of the philosophy of Kant and Hegel and the romantic spirit of the time—the emphasis on will and morale—to which they had been much attracted in their youth. Later Marxists also praised the German strategist. (Section IC, 1-5.)

In the following section, we see Trotsky delighting in demonstrating that the young Soviet military theorist, Michael Frunze's so-called 'proletarian' strategy was the same as that of the eighteenth-century Tsarist general, Suvarov, and that the supposedly 'Marxist' strategy of attack had been set forth by the French Marshal Foch, with disastrous results, in the early years of the First World War. Frunze and his supporters had cited the military 'theory' of the *Anti-Dühring* in opposition to Trotsky's empiricism. An unrepentant Trotsky replied that the method chosen by the Soviets to fight against the White Army was not derived from Marxist doctrine as Frunze insisted, but grew out of the character of a civil war, and the backwardness of Russian society and the Red Army. When these conditions changed, the military methods would change. (Section ID, 1a-b.) The leading Soviet military academy is named after Frunze.

Mao Tse-Tung (1893-1976), the Hunan-born leader of the Chinese Communist party, was the military organizer and strategist of the victory of its Red Army over the Nationalist forces in a lengthy civil war which ended in 1949. Like Trotsky, Mao fought against the doctrinaire views of a left-group of Marxist strategists, though, as we shall see later, he himself was to create a new version of the Marxist 'science' of war. In this selection, Mao displayed an apparently un-Marxist insistence that it was not weapons (i.e. technology) but people, and their morale, which were the decisive factors in war. (Section

IE.) Of course, such a view on Mao's part is understandable since otherwise the peasantry of the under-developed nations would have no chance of victory against the superior technology of the advanced, 'imperialist' powers. As we shall observe in subsequent selections (e.g. Section VF, G), this Clausewitzian opinion is shared by Soviet theorists as well.

Recent Soviet military theorists have made much of the usefulness of the dialectical method which Marx derived from Hegel—of understanding the movement from thesis to antithesis and the final resolution of this contradiction in a synthesis—in the determination of all military questions. In the last selection of this section, we have a eulogy of the effectiveness of this philosophical method in the construction of a Marxist military science. (Section IF.) In a later selection (Section VE), we will see how Soviet theorists have attempted a more practical application of this method.

Colonel V. Y. Savkin has served as a member of the faculty of the élite Frunze Military Academy. A review of his *Basic Principles of Operational Art and Tactics* (1972), which appeared in the Soviet military journal *Red Star*, in April 1973, made special mention of the properly Marxist–Leninist character of Savkin's discussion of the military theorists of the past. Colonel Savkin designed this work to discuss practical military problems 'from a position of Marxist–Leninist philosophy' for the benefit of 'officers and generals of the Soviet Army'. He is also known as the author of studies of the rate of advance in modern combat.

Colonels B. Byely and G. Fyodorov, and Captain V. Kulakov headed a team of fifteen army officers in an examination of how 'the basic principles of teaching on war and the army were worked out by Karl Marx and Friedrich Engels and were developed by Lenin.' These principles constitute 'a harmonious sociological teaching', the writers announced, adding that 'the method of dialectical materialism makes it possible to foresee the future scientifically.' The book has gone through several editions, and has been used in the academies which train Soviet army and navy officers. (See also selections from Byely and his colleagues in Sections III and V.) Parts of Section IF display the somewhat ritualistic character of the appeal to dialectics.

IA. Engels, 'The Force Theory'*

But let us look a little more closely at this omnipotent 'force' of Herr Dühring's. Crusoe enslaved Friday 'sword in hand.' Where did he get the sword from? Even on the imaginary islands of Crusoe stories, swords have not, up to now, grown on trees, and Herr Dühring gives us no answer whatever to this question. Just as Crusoe could procure a sword for himself, we are equally entitled to assume that one fine morning Friday might appear with a loaded revolver in his hand, and then the whole 'force' relationship is inverted. Friday commands, and it is Crusoe who has to drudge. We must apologise to the readers for returning with such insistence to the Crusoe and Friday story, which properly belongs to the nursery and not to science—but how can we help it? We are compelled to apply Herr Dühring's axiomatic method conscientiously, and it is not our fault if in doing so we have to keep all the time within the field of pure childishness. So, then, the revolver triumphs over the sword; and this will probably make even the most childish axiomatician comprehend that force is no mere act of the will, but requires very real preliminary conditions before it can come into operation, that is to say, *instruments*, the more perfect of which vanquish the less perfect; moreover, that these instruments have to be produced, which also implies that the producer of more perfect instruments of force, *vulgo* arms, vanquishes the producer of the less perfect instrument, and that, in a word, the triumph of force is based on the production of arms, and this in turn on production in general—therefore, on 'economic power,' on the 'economic order,' on the *material* means which force has at its disposal.

Force, nowadays, is the army and navy, and both, as we all know to our cost, are 'devilishly expensive.' Force, however, cannot make any money; at most it can only take away money that has already been made—and even this does not help very much—as we have seen, also to our cost, in the case of the French milliards. In the last analysis, therefore, money must be provided through the medium of economic production; and so once again force is conditioned by the economic order, which furnishes the resources for the equipment and main-

* Friedrich Engels, *Anti-Dühring; Herr Eugen Dühring's Revolution in Science* (1878), Part II, Chapter III.

tenance of the instruments of force. But even that is not all. Nothing is more dependent on economic pre-conditions than precisely the army and navy. Their armaments, composition, organisation, tactics and strategy depend above all on the stage reached at the time in production and communciations. It is not the 'free creations of the mind' of generals of genius which have revolutionised war, but the invention of better weapons and changes in the human material, the soldiers; at the very most, the part played by generals of genius is limited to adapting methods of fighting to the new weapons and combatants.

At the beginning of the fourteenth century, gunpowder came from the Arabs to Western Europe, and, as every school child knows, completely revolutionised methods of warfare. The introduction of gunpowder and firearms, however, was not at all an act of force, but a step forward in industry, that is, an economic advance. Industry remains industry, whether it is applied to the production or the destruction of things. And the introduction of firearms had a revolutionising effect not only on the waging of war itself, but also on the political relationships of domination and subjection. The provision of powder and firearms required industry and money, and both of these were in the hands of the burghers of the towns. From the outset, therefore, firearms were the weapons of the towns, and of the rising monarchy drawing its support from the towns, against the feudal nobility. The stone walls of the nobleman's castles, hitherto unapproachable, fell before the cannon of the burghers, and the bullets of the burghers' arquebuses pierced the armour of the knights. With the armour-clad cavalry of the feudal lords, the feudal lords' supremacy was also broken; with the development of the bourgeoisie, infantry and guns became more and more the decisive types of weapons; compelled by the development of artillery, the military profession had to add to its organisation a new and entirely industrial sub-section, the corps of engineers.

The improvement of firearms was a very slow process. Artillery remained clumsy and the musket, in spite of a number of inventions affecting details, was still a crude weapon. It took over three hundred years before a weapon was constructed which was suitable for the equipment of the whole body of infantry. It was not until the early part of the eighteenth century that the flint-lock musket with a bayonet finally displaced the pike in the equipment of the infantry. The foot soldiers of that period were the mercenaries of princes; they consisted of the most demoralised elements of society, rigorously disciplined, but quite unreliable and only held together by the whip; they were often enemy prisoners of war who had been pressed into service. The only type of fighting in which these soldiers could apply the new weapons was the tactics of the line, which reached its highest perfection under Frederick II. The whole infantry of an army was drawn up in triple ranks in the form of a very long, hollow square, and moved in battle order as a whole; at very most, one or other of the two wings might move forward or withdraw a little. This cumbrous mass could only move in formation on absolutely level ground, and even then only at a very slow rate (seventy-five paces a minute); a change of formation during a battle was impossible, and once the infantry was engaged, victory or defeat was decided rapidly and at a single blow.

In the American War of Independence, these cumbrous lines came up against bands of insurgents, which although not drilled were all the better able to shoot from their rifled carbines; these rebels were fighting for their own special interests, and therefore did not desert like the mercenaries; nor did they do the English the kindness of advancing against them also in line and across the open plain, but in scattered and rapidly moving troops of sharpshooters under cover of the woods. In such circumstances the line was powerless and was defeated by its invisible and intangible opponents. Fighting in skirmishing order was re-invented—a new method of warfare which was the result of a change in the human material of war.

In the military sphere also, the French Revolution completed what the American Revolution had begun. Like the American, the French Revolution could oppose to the trained mercenary armies of the coalition only poorly trained but great masses of soldiers, the levy of the whole nation. But these masses had to protect Paris, that is, to hold a definite area, and for this purpose victory in open battle on a mass scale was essential. Mere skirmishes did not suffice; a form had to be invented for use by large bodies of troops, and this form was found in the *column*. Column formation made it possible for even poorly trained troops to move with a fair degree of order, and moreover with greater speed (a hundred paces and more in a minute); it made it possible to break through the rigid forms of the old line formation; to fight on any ground, and therefore even on ground which was extremely disadvantageous to the line formation; to group the troops in any appropriate way; and, in conjunction with attacks by scattered bands of sharpshooters, to hold up the enemy's lines, keeping them occupied and wearing them out until the moment came for masses held in reserve to break through them at the decisive point in the position. This new method of warfare, based on the combined action of skirmishers and columns and on the partitioning of the army into independent divisions or army corps, composed of all types of arms—a method brought to full perfection by Napoleon in both its tactical and strategical aspects—had become necessary primarily because of the changed material: the soldiery of the French Revolution. But it also had two other very important preliminary technical conditions: first, the lighter carriages for field guns constructed by Gribeauval, which alone made possible the more rapid movement now required of them; and secondly, the slanting of the butt, which had hitherto been quite straight, continuing the line of the barrel; introduced in France in 1777, it was copied from hunting weapons and it made it possible to shoot at an individual man without necessarily missing him. But for this improvement it would have been impossible to adopt skirmishing tactics, for which the old weapons were useless.

The revolutionary system of arming the whole people was soon restricted to compulsory conscription (with substitution for the rich, by payment of money) and in this form it was adopted by most of the large states on the Continent. Only Prussia attempted, through its *Landwehr* system, to draw to a still greater extent on the defensive power of the people. After the rifled muzzle-loader, which had been improved between 1830 and 1860 and made suitable for use in war, had played a brief role, Prussia was also the first state to equip its whole infantry with the most up-to-date weapons, the rifled breech-loader. Its successes in 1866 were due to these two factors.

The Franco-Prussian War was the first in which two armies

faced each other both equipped with breech-loading rifles, and moreover both fundamentally in the same tactical formations as in the time of the old smooth-bore flint-locks. The only difference was that the Prussians had introduced the company column formation in an attempt to find a form of fighting which was better adapted to the new type of arms. But when, at St. Privat on August 18, the Prussian Guard tried to apply the company column formation seriously, the five regiments which were chiefly engaged lost in less than two hours more than a third of their strength (176 officers and 5,114 men). From that time the company column formation too was condemned, no less than the battalion column and the line; all idea of exposing troops in any kind of closed formation to enemy gunfire was abandoned, and on the German side all subsequent fighting was conducted only in those compact bodies of skirmishers into which the columns had so far regularly dissolved of themselves under a deadly hail of bullets, although this had been opposed by the higher officers on the ground that it was contrary to good discipline; and in the same way the only form of movement when under fire from enemy rifles became the *double*. Once again the soldier had been shrewder than the officer; it was he who instinctively found the only way of fighting which has proved of service up to now under the fire of breech-loading rifles, and in spite of opposition from his officers he carried it through successfully.

The Franco-Prussian War marked a turning-point which was of entirely new significance. In the first place the weapons used have reached such a stage of perfection that further progress which would have any revolutionising influence is no longer possible. Once armies have guns which can hit a battalion at any range at which it can be distinguished, and rifles which are equally effective for hitting individual men, while loading them takes less time than aiming, then all further improvements are more or less unimportant for field warfare. The era of evolution is therefore, in essentials, closed in this direction. And secondly, this war compelled all continental Powers to introduce in a stricter form the Prussian *Landwehr* system, and with it a military burden which must bring them to ruin within a few years. The army has become the main purpose of the state, and an end in itself; the peoples are only there in addition in order to provide and feed the soldiers. Militarism dominates and is swallowing Europe. But this militarism also carries in itself the seed of its own destruction. Competition of the individual states with each other forces them, on the one hand, to spend more money each year on the army and navy, artillery, etc., thus more and more hastening financial catastrophe; and on the other hand, to take universal compulsory military service more and more seriously, thus in the long run making the whole people familiar with the use of arms; and therefore making the people more and more able at a given moment to make its will prevail in opposition to the commanding military lords. And this moment comes as soon as the mass of the people—town and country workers and peasants—*has* a will. At this point the armies of princes become transformed into armies of the people; the machine refuses to work, and militarism collapses by the dialectic of its own evolution. What the bourgeois democracy of 1848 could not accomplish, just because it was *bourgeois* and not proletarian, namely, to give the labouring masses a will whose content was in accord with their class position—socialism will infallibly secure. And this will mean the bursting asunder of militarism *from within*, and with it of all standing armies.

That is the first moral of our history of modern infantry. The second moral, which brings us back again to Herr Dühring, is that the whole organisation and method of fighting of armies, and along with these victory or defeat, proves to be dependent on material, that is, economic conditions; on the human material, and the armaments material, and therefore on the quality and quantity of the population and on technical development. Only a hunting people like the Americans could re-discover skirmishing tactics—and they were hunters as a result of purely economic causes, just as now, as a result of purely economic causes, these same Yankees of the old States have been transformed into farmers, industrialists, seamen and merchants who no longer skirmish in the primeval forests, but instead skirmish all the more effectively on the field of speculation, where they have made considerable progress with it also in its mass application. Only a revolution such as the French, which brought about the economic emancipation of the burghers and especially of the peasantry, could find the method of the mass army and at the same time the free form of movement which shattered the old rigid lines—the military counterparts of the absolutism against which they were fighting. And we have seen in case after case how advances in technique, as soon as they became usable in the military sphere and in fact were so used, immediately and almost violently produced changes in the methods of warfare and indeed revolutionised them, often even against the will of the army command. And nowadays any zealous subaltern could explain to Herr Dühring how greatly the conduct of a war depends on the productivity and means of communication of the army's own hinterland as well as of the arena of war. In short, always and everywhere it is the economic conditions and instruments of force which help 'force' to victory, and without these, force ceases to be force. And anyone who tried to reform methods of warfare from the opposite standpoint, on the basis of Dühringian principles, would certainly reap nothing but a beating.*

If we pass now from land to sea, even in the last twenty years we find a complete revolution of quite a different order. The warship of the Crimean war was the wooden two and three-decker of 60 to 100 guns; these were still mainly sailing ships, with only a low-powered auxiliary steam engine. The guns on these warships were for the most part 32-pounders weighing approximately 2½ tons, with a few 68-pounders weighing approximately 4¾ tons. Towards the end of the war, iron-clad floating batteries made their appearance; they were clumsy and almost immobile, but to the guns of that period they were invulnerable monsters. Soon the iron armour plating was applied also to warships; at first the plates were still very thin, a ship with plates four inches thick being regarded as extremely heavily armoured. But soon the progress made with artillery outstripped the armour-plating; each successive increase in the strength of the armour used was countered by a new and heavier gun which easily pierced the plates. In this

* This is already perfectly well known to the Prussian General Staff. 'The *basis* of warfare is primarily the general *economic* life of the peoples.' This was said in a scientific lecture by Herr Marx Jähns, a captain of the General Staff. (*Kölnische Zeitung*, April 20, 1876, p. 3.) [*Note by F. Engels.*]

way we have already reached armour-plating ten, twelve, fourteen and twenty-four inches in thickness (Italy proposes to build a ship with plates three feet thick) on the one hand, and on the other, rifled guns of 25, 35, 80 and even 100 tons in weight, which can hurl projectiles, weighing 300, 400, 1,700 and up to 2,000 pounds to distances which were never dreamed of before. The warship of the present day is a gigantic armoured screw-driven vessel of 8,000 to 9,000 tons and 6,000 to 8,000 horse power, with revolving turrets and four or at most six heavy guns and with a bow extended under water into a ram for running down enemy vessels; it is a single colossal machine, in which steam not only drives the ship at a high speed, but also works the steering-gear, raises the anchor, swings the turrets, changes the elevation of the guns and loads them, pumps out water, hoists and lowers the boats—some of which are themselves also steam driven—and so forth. And the rivalry between armour-plating and the efficacy of guns is so far from being at an end that nowadays a ship is almost always not up to requirements, already out of date, before it is launched. The modern warship is not only a product, but at the same time a specimen of modern large-scale industry, a floating factory—producing mainly, to be sure, a lavish waste of money. The country in which large-scale industry is most highly developed has almost a monopoly in the construction of these ships. All Turkish, almost all Russian and most German armoured vessels are built in England; serviceable armour-plates are hardly made outside of Sheffield; of the three steel works in Europe which alone are able to make the heaviest guns, two (Woolwich and Elswick) are in England, and the third (Krupp) in Germany. In this sphere it is most palpably evident that the 'direct political force' which, according to Herr Dühring, is the 'determining cause of the economic order,' is on the contrary completely subordinated to the economic order; that not only the construction but also the manipulation of the marine instrument of force, the warship, has itself become a branch of modern large-scale industry. And that this is so distresses no one more than force itself, that is, the state, which has now to pay for one ship as much as a whole fleet used to cost; which has to resign itself to seeing these expensive vessels becoming already out of date, and therefore worthless, before they get into the water; and which must certainly be just as disgusted as Herr Dühring that the man of the 'economic order, the engineer, is now of far greater importance on board than the man of 'direct force,' the captain. We on the contrary have absolutely no cause for annoyance when we see that, in this competitive struggle between armour-plating and guns, the warship is being developed to a pitch of perfection which is making it both outrageously costly and unusable in war,* and that this struggle makes manifest also in the sphere of naval warfare those immanent dialectical laws of motion on the basis of which militarism, like all other historical phenomena, is being brought to destruction as a result of its own development.

Here too, therefore, we see absolutely clearly that it is not in any way true 'the primitive phenomenon must be sought in direct political force and not in any indirect economic power.' On the contrary. For what in fact does 'the primitive' in force itself prove to be? Economic power, control over the means of force in large-scale industry. Political naval power which is dependent on modern warships, proves to be not at all 'direct' but on the contrary *conditioned* by economic power, the high development of metallurgy, and the command of skilled technicians and productive coal mines.

And yet what is the use of it all? If we put Herr Dühring in supreme comand in the next naval war, he will utterly destroy all fleets of armoured ships which are slaves of the economic order, without torpedoes or any other artifices, by sole virture of his 'direct force'.

IB. Trotsky, 'On Marxism and Military Science'

1.†

Up to now we have successfully coped with the military tasks imposed upon us by the international and domestic position

* The perfecting of the latest production of large-scale industry for use in naval warfare, the self-propelling torpedo, seems likely to bring this to pass; it would mean that the smallest torpedo-boat would be superior to the most powerful armoured battle-ship. [Note by F. Engels.]

† Excerpts from L. Trotsky, 'Military Doctrine or Pseudo-Military Doctrinairism', Dec. 5 1921, *Military Writings* (New York, 1969), pp. 32 ff.

of Soviet Russia. Our orientation proved to be more correct, more farsighted and deeper-going than the orientation of the mightiest imperialist powers who have sought individually and collectively to bring us down, but who burned their fingers in the attempt. Our superiority lies in possessing the irreplaceable scientific method of orientation—Marxism. It is the most powerful and at the same time subtle instrument—to use it is not as easy as shelling peas. One must learn how to operate with it. Our party's past has taught us through long and hard experience just how to apply the methods of Marxism to the most complex combination of factors and forces during the historical epoch of sharpest breaks. We likewise employ the instrument of Marxism in order to define the basis for our military construction.

It is quite otherwise with our enemies. If the advanced bourgeoisie has banished inertia, routinism and superstition from the domain of productive technology, and has sought to build each enterprise on the precise foundations of scientific methods, then in the field of social orientation the bourgeoisie has proved impotent, because of its class position, to rise to the heights of scientific method. Our class enemies are empiricists, that is, they operate from one occasion to the next, guided not by the analysis of historical development, but by practical experience, routinism, rule of the thumb, and instinct. . . .

If it may be said of the most far-sighted empiricists of English imperialism that they have a key-ring with a considerable variety of keys good for *many* typical historical situations, then we hold in our hands a universal key which does us service in *all* situations. And while the entire supply of keys inherited by Lloyd George, Churchill and the others is obviously no good for opening a way out of the revolutionary epoch, our Marxist key is predestined above all for this purpose. We are not afraid to speak aloud about this, our greatest advantage over our adversaries, for they are impotent to acquire or to counterfeit our Marxist key.

We foresaw the inevitability of the imperialist war as the prologue to the epoch of proletarian revolution. With this as our starting point we then kept following the course of the war, the methods employed in it, the shifts in the groupings of class forces and on the basis of our observations there crystallized much more directly—if one were to employ a pompous style—the 'doctrine' of the Soviet system and the Red Army. From the scientific foresight of the further course of events we gained unconquerable confidence that history is working in our favor. And this optimistic confidence has been and remains the foundation of all our activity.

*IB, 2.**

What is the Marxist method? It is a method of thinking scientifically. It is the method of historical social science. True enough, our army magazine bears the name: *Military Science.* But our magazine still contains many incongruities left over from the past, and most incongruous of all is its name. There is not and there never has been a military 'science.' There does exist a whole number of sciences upon which military affairs rest. Included among them essentially are all the sciences from geography to psychology: An outstanding army leader must possess the knowledge of the elementary principles of many sciences—although, to be sure, there are self-taught army leaders who act on the basis of probing empirically, but who are assisted by a certain innate sense. War rests on many sciences, but war itself is not a science—it is a practical art, a skill. The Prussian strategist, King Frederick II was fond of saying that war is a trade for an ignoramus, an art for a man of talent and a science for a genius. But he told a lie. This is false. For an ignoramus war is not a trade because ignorant soldiers are the cannon fodder of war and not at all its 'tradesmen.' As is well known, each trade requires a certain schooling; and for those who are correctly schooled in military affairs war is therefore a 'trade.' It is a cruel, sanguinary trade, but a trade nonetheless, that is, a skill with certain habits which are elaborated by experience and correctly assimilated. For gifted people and those of genius, this skill becomes transformed into a high art.

War cannot be turned into a science because of its very nature, no more than it is possible to turn architecture, commerce or a veterinary's occupation into a science. What is

* Excerpts from L. Trotsky, 'Our Current Basic Military Tasks', April 1 1922, *Military Writings*, pp. 72–5.

commonly called the theory of war or military science represents not a totality of scientific laws explaining objective events but an aggregate of practical usages, methods of adaptation and proficiencies corresponding to a specific task: the task of crushing the enemy. Whoever masters these usages to a high degree and on a broad scale and is able to attain great results by means of combinations—such an individual raises military affairs to the level of a cruel and sanguinary *art.* But there is no ground whatever to talk of science here. Our statutes are just a compilation of the practical rules derived from experience.

Marxism on the other hand is a method of science, that is, the science of apprehending objective events in their objective connections. Just how is it possible to construct the usages of a military trade or art by means of the Marxist method? This is the same thing as trying to construct a theory of architecture or a text book on veterinary medicine with the aid of the Marxist method. A history of war, like a history of architecture can be written from the Marxist viewpoint, because history is a science. But a so-called theory of war, i.e., practical [military] leadership is something else again. These must not be mixed up, otherwise the result is not a unified world-outlook but the greatest muddle.

With the aid of the Marxist method, social-political and international orientation is facilitated in the extreme. This is incontestable. Only with the aid of Marxism is it possible to analyze the world situation, especially in our modern and exceptional epoch.

But it is impossible to construct a field statute with the aid of Marxism. The blunder here lies in interpreting military doctrine or, what is worse, 'unified military world-outlook' to include our general state orientation, both international and internal, as well as practical military usages, statute regulations and precepts—with the expressed desire of seemingly rebuilding all this anew with the aid of the Marxist method. . . .

It turns out [according to Frunze] that our military system derives wholly from the specific class nature of the proletarian state. Presumably the task is first to determine this nature, next deduce from it a unified military doctrine, and then obtain from the latter all the necessary partial, practical conclusions. This method is scholastic and hopeless. The class nature of the proletarian state determines the social composition of the Red Army and particularly of its leading apparatus; it determines its political world-outlook, its aims and its moods. Naturally, all this exerts a certain indirect influence upon strategy and tactics alike, and yet strategy and tactics are not derived from a proletarian world-outlook but from the conditions of technology, in particular military technology, from the available facilities of providing supplies, from the geographical milieu, the character of the enemy, etc., etc.

Do we possess a unified industrial or a unified commercial world-outlook? Is it possible for us to deduce from the 'specific nature of the proletarian state' the best textbook of foreign trade, or the best method of administrative or commercial organization for our trusts? An attempt to do this would be ludicrous and hopeless. To think that by arming oneself with the Marxist method it is possible to solve the question of how best to organize production in a candle factory, is to understand nothing either about the Marxist method or about a candle factory. Meanwhile, an army regiment from the standpoint of its own specific tasks is a factory that must be correctly organized, that is, in harmony with its purposes. I assert that an attempt to derive from the system of the proletarian state by means of deduction, i.e. logically, the organization, structure, and tactical usages of an infantry or cavalry regiment is absolutely utopian and nonsensical.

*IB, 3.**

Military science does not belong among natural sciences, because it is neither 'natural' nor a 'science.' Our discussion today may perhaps bring us closer to clarification on this question.

But even if one grants that 'military science' is a *science*, it is nevertheless impossible to grant that it can be built with the methods of Marxism; because historical materialism isn't at all a universal method for all sciences. This is the greatest possible misconception which, it seems to me, can lead to the most harmful consequences. It is possible to devote an entire

* Excerpts from L. Trotsky, 'Marxism and Military Knowledge', May 8 1922, *Military Writings*, pp. 110–13, 116 f., 119 ff.

lifetime to military affairs very successfully, without ever devoting any thought to theoretical-epistemological methods in military matters—just as I am able to take daily readings of my watch without knowing anything about its internal workings, its interplay of wheels and levers. . . .

In the course of a previous discussion (on unified military doctrine) I adduced one of the traits of George V. Plekhanov, the first crusader for Marxism on Russian soil, a man of broad vision and high gifts. Whenever Plekhanov observed that questions of philosophic materialism and historical materialism were being opposed to one another, or on the contrary lumped together, he hotly protested. Philosophic materialism is a theory imbedded in the foundation of *natural* sciences; while historical materialism explains the history of *human society*. Historical materialism is a method that explains not the structure of the entire universe, but a rigidly *delimited* group of phenomena; a method that analyzes the development of historical man. Philosophic materialism explains the movement of the universe as matter in the process of change and transformation; and it extends its explanation to include the 'highest' manifestation of the spirit. It is difficult, if not impossible, to be a Marxist in politics and remain ignorant of historical materialism. It is quite possible to be a Marxist in politics and not know about philosophic materialism; such instances can be adduced to any number. . . .

My premise is that we should follow in the excellent tradition of the deceased Plekhanov in the field of applying philosophy to military affairs. We are not at all obliged to occupy ourselves with questions which are known as 'gnosiological,' 'theoretical-epistemological,' philosophical; but once we do take them up, then it is impermissible to muddle, and to go wandering with wrong instruments into an entirely different field in the attempt to apply the method of Marxism directly to military affairs, in the proper meaning of this word (not military politics).

It is the greatest misconception to try to build in the special sphere of military matters by means of the method of Marxism; no less a misconception is the attempt to include military matters in the list of natural sciences. . . .

So far as our today's session is concerned, the benefits of

discussing the broad question of the relation between military affairs and Marxism will be rather those, so to speak, of mental hygiene: There will be less confusion. And in practical terms our task is: Let us learn to speak more simply about the cavalry; let us not clutter up our discussion of aviation with ostentatious Marxist terminology, high-sounding terms, pompous problems which turn out, one and all, to be hollow shells without kernel or content. . . .

For philosophic terminology is an artifice akin to make-up. . . . The make-up may be terribly imposing but underneath it there is nothing at all. Yet, as I have had occasion to note from many articles in our military publications, this occultism for the augurs, this occult procedure for the initiated, these medieval traditions and practices are retained among us. And so, I ask you to expound your ideas as simply as possible. . . .

What is trade—a science or an art? Marx made a science out of trade—in the sense that he established the laws of capitalist society, he made trade the object of scientific investigation. But can one trade 'according to Marx'? No, this is impossible. One of the most stable, if not eternal principles of trade is the rule: 'No cheating, no sale.' Marxism explains whence arose this 'principle' and how it later came to be supplanted by Italian double bookkeeping, which expresses the self-same thing but in a more delicate way. But is Marxism able to create a new system of bookkeeping? Or is a Marxist freed of the necessity of studying bookkeeping if he seriously wishes to take up trading? Behind the attempts to proclaim Marxism as the method of all sciences and arts there frequently lurks a stubborn refusal to enter new fields. For it is much easier to possess a '*passe-partout*,' that is, a master key that opens all doors and locks, rather than study bookkeeping, military affairs, etc. This is the greatest danger in all attempts to invest the Marxist method with such an absolute character. Marx attacked such pseudo-Marxists. In one of his letters he literally said, 'I am no Marxist,' when in place of an explanation of the historical process, in place of a careful and conscientious investigation of what was occurring Marx was proffered some kind of itinerary for history. Even less did Marx intend to replace all other fields of human knowledge by his social-historical theory. Does this mean that a military leader has no need of the Marxist method? Not at all. It would be absurd to deny the great importance of materialism for disciplining the mind in all fields. Marxism, like Darwinism, is the highest school of human thought. Methods of warfare cannot be deduced from Darwin's theory, from the law of natural selection; but an army leader who studied Darwin would be, given other qualifications, better equipped. He would have a wider horizon and be more fertile in devices; he would take note of those aspects of nature and man which previously had passed unnoticed. This applies to Marxism even to a greater extent. . . .

It is absolutely correct that a historical point of view is fruitful in the extreme and that a history of science is superior to any Kantian epistemology. . . . Terms must be approached *historically*. But a history of terms, hypotheses and theories does not replace science itself. Physics is physics. Military affairs are military affairs. . . .

An aggregate of 'military principles' does not constitute a military science, for there is no more a science of war than there is a science of locksmithing. An army leader requires the knowledge of a whole number of sciences in order to feel himself fully equipped for his *art.* But military science does not exist; there does exist a military craft which can be raised to the level of military art.

A scientific history of warfare is not military science but social science, or a branch of social science. A scientific history of warfare explains why in a given epoch, with a given social organization, men waged war in a certain way and not differently; and why such and such usages led in this epoch to victory whereas other methods brought defeat. Beginning with the general condition of productive forces, a scientific history of war must take into account all the superstructural factors, even the furthest removed, including the plans and the mistakes of the commanding staff. But it is quite self-evident that a scientific history of war aims by its very nature to explain that which undergoes change and the reasons for these changes, but not to establish eternal truths.

What truths can history give us? The role and significance of the growth of medieval cities in the development of military affairs. The invention of firearms. The overthrow of the feudal system and the significance of this revolution with respect to the army, and so on.

Marxist political economy is an incontestable science; but it is not a science of how to manage a business, or how to compete on the market, or how to build trusts. It is the science of how in a certain epoch certain economic relations (capitalist) took shape, and what conditions these relations internally, and constitutes their lawfulness. Economic laws established by Marx are not eternal truths but characteristic only of a specific epoch of mankind's economic development; and, in any case, they are not eternal principles as is represented by the bourgeois Manchester school, according to which private ownership of the means of production, buying and selling, competition and the rest are eternal principles of economy, deriving from human nature (about which however there is absolutely nothing eternal)....

Doctrinaires in military affairs behave in exactly the same way with regard to military truths. Military generalizations, or more correctly the usages of a certain epoch, are transformed by them into eternal truths. If people were previously unaware of these eternal truths, so much the worse for those who wallowed in the mire of barbarism. But ever since their discovery, they remain eternal principles of military affairs.... The army of *landsknechts*, the regular armies of the seventeenth and eighteenth centuries, the national army called to life by the Great French Revolution—all these correspond to definite epochs of economic and political development, and they all rest upon a certain technology on which they depend for their structure and methods of operation. Military history can and must establish this social conditioning of the army and its methods. But what does military philosophy do? As a rule it looks upon the methods and usages of a preceding epoch as eternal truths, at last discovered by mankind and destined to retain their meaning for all times and all peoples. The discovery of these eternal truths is linked primarily with the Napoleonic epoch. The same truths and principles are then discovered in the operations of Hannibal and Caesar. The period of the Middle Ages is turned into a hiatus in the course of which the eternal principles of war were forgotten along with the science and philosophy of antiquity.

There is, however, a difference between the mistakes of Manchesterism and the mistakes of the doctrinaires of eternal principles of military science. This difference lies in the difference between the two kinds of activity. Economic relations in capitalist society take shape, as Marx said, behind people's backs, arising from their ant-like economic labors; and the people then find themselves confronted with already crystallized property relations which determine the relations between man and man.

In military affairs the element of planned construction, of conscious direction by the human will comes into play on a far greater scope. Under capitalist relations plan, will, calculation, supervision, initiative are applied within the limits of an individual economy; and the laws of capitalist economy grow out of the relations between these individual economies: that is why they take shape 'behind the backs' of people. But the army is by its very nature an all-state enterprise and consequently plans and projects are here applied within a state framework. This does not of course cancel the decisive dependence of military matters upon economy, but the subjective element in the person of military leaders attains a scope which cannot obtain in the sphere of economy. . . .

IC. The Case of Clausewitz

1. Engels and Marx on Clausewitz

*a.** I'm now reading, among other things, Clausewitz's *On War*. An extraordinary way of philosophizing on these matters, but very good. On the question as to whether one ought to speak of the Art of War or the Science of War, his answer is that war is most like Commerce. Fighting is in war what cash payment is in trade, as seldom as it may in reality need to take place, everything is directed toward it, and in the end it must occur and decide the issue.

*b.*** On the occasion of writing my article on Blücher, I did some general reading of Clausewitz. The chap has a *common sense* that borders on brilliance.

* Engels to Marx (Jan. 7 1858), *Marx-Engels Werke* (Berlin: Dietz Verlag, 1963), XXIX, 252.

** Marx to Engels (Jan. 11 1858), *Marx-Engels Werke*, XXIX, 256.

*IC, 2. Lenin on Clausewitz**

'WAR IS THE CONTINUATION OF POLITICS BY OTHER (I.E.: VIOLENT) MEANS'

This famous dictum was uttered by Clausewitz, one of the profoundest writers on the problems of war. Marxists have always rightly regarded this thesis as the theoretical basis of views on the significance of any war. It was from this viewpoint that Marx and Engels always regarded the various wars.

Apply this view to the present war. You will see that for decades, for almost half a century, the governments and the ruling classes of Britain and France, Germany and Italy, Austria and Russia have pursued a policy of plundering colonies, oppressing other nations, and suppressing the working-class movement. It is this, and only this, policy that is being continued in the present war. In particular, the policy of both Austria and Russia, in peacetime as well as in wartime, is a policy of enslaving nations, not of liberating them. In China, Persia, India and other dependent countries, on the contrary, we have seen during the past decades a policy of rousing tens and hundreds of millions of people to a national life, of their liberation from the reactionary 'Great' Powers' oppression. A war waged on such a historical basis can even today be a bourgeois-progressive war of national liberation.

If the present war is regarded as a continuation of the politics of the 'Great' Powers and of the principal classes within them, a glance will immediately reveal the glaring antihistoricity, falseness and hypocrisy of the view that the 'defence-of-the-fatherland' idea can be justified in the present war.

*IC, 3. Trotsky on Clausewitz***

According to the traditional point of view, the foundations of military science are eternal and common to all times and all peoples. But in their concrete refraction these eternal truths assume a national character. Hence are derived: the German military doctrine, the French military doctrine, the

* V. I. Lenin, 'Socialism and War' (1915), *Collected Works* (Moscow, 1964-5), XXI: 304 f.

** Excerpts from L. Trotsky, 'Military Doctrine or Pseudo-Military Doctrinairism', Dec. 5 1921, *Military Writings*, pp. 38, 42 f., 56 f.

Russian military doctrine, and so forth and so on. But if we check the inventory of the eternal truths of military science we obtain little from them beyond a few logical axioms and Euclidian postulates. The flanks must be defended; the means of communication and retreat must be secured; the blow must be directed at the opponent's least defended point, etc., etc. In their essence all these truths, in this all-embracing formulation, transcend far beyond the limits of military art. A donkey in pilfering oats from a torn sack (the opponent's least defended point) and at the same time in turning its rump vigilantly away from the side from which danger may threaten, acts on the basis of the eternal principles of military science. Meanwhile, it is unquestionable that this donkey munching oats has never read Clausewitz.

War, the subject of our discussion, is a social and historical phenomenon which arises, develops, changes its forms and must eventually disappear. For this reason alone war cannot have any eternal laws. The subject of war is man who possesses certain stable anatomical and psychical traits from which flow certain usages and habits. Man operates in a specific and relatively stable geographical milieu. Thus in all wars, during all times and among all peoples there have obtained certain common, relatively stable (but by no means absolute) traits. Based on these traits there has developed historically a military art. Its methods and usages undergo change together with the social conditions which determine it (technology, class structure, forms of state power). . . .

Only the Marxist method of international orientation, of calculating the class forces in all their combinations and shifts can enable us to find a proper solution in each given concrete case. It is impossible to invent a general formula that would express the 'essence' of our military tasks in the next period.

One can, however—and this is not infrequently done—endow the concept of military doctrine with a far more concrete and narrow content, by restricting its meaning to those elementary principles of purely military affairs which regulate all the aspects of military organization, tactics and strategy. In this sense it may be said that the content of military statutes is determined directly by military doctrine. But what kind of principles are these? Certain doctrinaires depict the matter as follows: It is first necessary to establish the essence and purpose of the army and the task before it; from this definition one then derives the army's organization, its strategy and tactics; and incorporates these deductions in statutes. In reality, such an approach to the question is scholastic and lifeless.

An inkling of the assortment of banalities and idle chatter that are subsumed under the elementary principles of military art may be gleaned from the solemnly quoted statement of Foch to the effect that the essence of modern war consists in 'once the hostile armies are located in destroying them, employing to this end the direction and tactics which lead most quickly and surely to the desired goal.' How profound! What boundless horizons this opens before us! To amplify this one need only add that the essence of modern methods of nutrition consists in locating the aperture of the mouth, introducing food therein, and, after it has been masticated with the least possible expenditure of energy—in swallowing it. Why shouldn't one try to deduce from this principle—which is in no way inferior to that of Foch—precisely what the food is and how it must be prepared and just when and just who should swallow it; and, above all, how this food is to be procured.

Military affairs are very empirical, very practical affairs. It is a very risky exercise to attempt to erect them into a system from whose fundamental principles are to be deduced field statutes and the structure of squadrons and the cut of the uniform. This was very well understood by old Clausewitz who said:

> It is not impossible, perhaps, to write a systematic theory of war, both logical and wide in scope. But our theory, up to the present, is far from being either. Not to mention their unscientific spirit in the attempt to make their systems consistent and complete, many such works are stuffed with commonplaces and idle chatter of every kind. . . .

We must reject all attempts at building an absolute revolutionary strategy with the elements of our limited experience of three years of civil war during which army sections of a special quality engaged in combat under special conditions. Clausewitz has warned very correctly against this. He wrote:

> What is more natural than that the revolutionary war (of France) had its own way of doing things? And what theory could have included

that peculiar method? The trouble is that such a manner, originating from a special case easily outlives its day, because it continues *unchanged* while circumstances imperceptibly undergo complete *change*. That is what theory should prevent by lucid and rational criticism. In 1806 the victims of this methodism were the Prussian generals . . .

Alas! The Prussian generals are not the only ones who incline toward methodism, i.e., platitudes and stereotypes.

*IC, 4. Byely on Clausewitz**

Clausewitz said that politics represents the interests of society as a whole, he denied its class nature. Accordingly he propounded a false, idealistic view of politics, which he called the mind of the personified state. Besides, Clausewitz understood by politics only foreign policy, and ignored the fact that war is first and foremost a continuation of domestic policy, which expresses the class structure of society most directly. Clausewitz had in mind only the politics of the state, that is, of the class dominant in the state in question. He did not believe that when the oppressed classes were fighting against the exploiters, they were thereby pursuing a policy of their own, and he therefore did not extend the concept of war to the civil wars of the popular masses against the exploiter classes and their state. Clausewitz completely ignored the fact that politics is conditioned by deep causes rooted in the economic system of society. . . .

In his remarks on Clausewitz's book *On War* Lenin wrote out, underlined and marked 'correct!' a proposition important to an understanding of the influence politics exerts on changes in the essence of war: '. . . war itself in its essence, in its forms has also undergone considerable changes . . . these changes emerged not because the French Government emancipated war, so to say, released it from the leash of politics—these changes emerged from the new politics that emerged from the womb of the French revolution not only for France, but also for the whole of Europe.'

Particularly deep changes in the interrelation between politics and war were introduced by the October Socialist Revolution, which overthrew the exploiter system in Russia,

* Excerpts from B. Byely, G. Fyodorov, V. Kulakov, *et al.*, *Marxism–Leninism on War and Army* (Moscow, 1972), pp. 16 f., 35 f.

put an end to the policy of social and national oppression which the exploiting classes were implementing, replaced it by a fundamentally different policy, by the qualitatively new political relations that emerged with the triumph of socialism. The revolutionary changes in politics had a major impact on the essence, content and character of the wars the Soviet state had to wage in self-defence. These wars were a continuation of the political struggle which the working people were waging for liberation from the capitalists in their own country and throughout the world.

*IC, 5. Savkin on Clausewitz**

Karl Clausewitz (1780-1831), the apex of German bourgeois military thought, also devotes much space to the principle of military art.

In Clausewitz, along with advanced thoughts and fierce criticism of the feudal military system, there lived side by side reactionary ideas which characterize him as a representative of Prussian military caste, with its militarism, nationalism, and antidemocratism. German idealism was the philosophical basis of Clausewitz's military theory, but Clausewitz's enormous advantage is the application of Hegel's dialectical method.

As a result of this, the philosophical basis of this theory was directed against dogmatism and metaphysics. . . .

In his chief work entitled *On War*, published in 1832-1834, Clausewitz draws the conclusion: 'One must commit the greatest number of troops possible at the decisive point.' the ratio of forces at the decisive point is an enormous matter, says Clausewitz, it is the most important of all the conditions. Here Clausewitz believed that in strategy the more force used the better, and that forces at one's disposal must be used simultaneously.

Clausewitz sometimes considered the achievement of surprise to be . . . the most important independent principle. It is obvious that he was correct in the last instance.

Clausewitz wrote . . . that once a major victory had been won, there must be no mention of rest or a breather; the agenda for the day is only pursuit and the delivery of new

* Excerpts from V. Ye. Savkin, *The Basic Principles of Operational Art and Tactics: A Soviet View* (US Air Force, 1972), pp. 22 ff.

strikes where necessary. In some chapters of his work Clausewitz defines activeness and decisiveness as an independent principle of military art. . . .

Clausewitz, whose ideas, in Lenin's words, 'were fertilized by Hegel, viewed the phenomena of war and military art in their development and movement, speaking out against 'eternal principles' of military art. Herein lies his service, but he erroneously denied the laws of military affairs or explained them idealistically, assuming that 'the conception of law in the sense of cognition in war is almost superfluous, since complex phenomena of war are insufficiently natural, and those which are natural are insufficiently complex.' Here Clausewitz proceeded from an assumption that war is the 'field of chance,' 'the field of the unauthentic: three-fourths of that on which action is built in warfare lies in the haze of obscurity.' From this comes an overestimation of the role of the general: 'Talent and genius operate outside the law,' and that which a genius does 'must be the best rule.'

Clausewitz's great service, which Lenin remarked on more than once, consists of establishment of the tie between war and politics.

This was a major achievement of military thinking of that time, in spite of the limitation of Clausewitz's formula and the fundamental distinction between Lenin's understanding of the essence of war and Clausewitz's viewpoint. Clausewitz denied the class nature of politics and understood politics to be only foreign policy, although in reality war is a continuation primarily of domestic policy, which directly reflects the class structure of society. He had in mind actually only the politics of the ruling class and did not recognize the presence of politics of the oppressed classes and the fact that politics was conditioned by the economic system of society.

ID. The Tradition and Marxist Military Doctrine

1. Trotsky surveys the tradition

a. 'The Principles of Foch'.* Von der Goltz, and after him Foch, acknowledged that the factors studied by military art

* L. Trotsky, 'Marxism and Military Knowledge', May 8 1922, *Military Writings,* pp. 124-32.

undergo change (the club, the musket, the automatic rifle, the machine gun, the cannon, and so on), but that the principles of the art remain if not eternal, then in any case unaltered since war first began.

What then are these principles? In his introduction to the second edition Foch seems to sponsor maneuverist offense as the main principle. But in the very first lecture he gives the following answer:

> 'And so, the theory of war exists. It puts to the fore the following principles:
> 'The principle of economy of forces.
> 'The principle of freedom of action.
> 'The principle of free disposition of forces.
> 'The principle of security.'

And so on.

And further, in order to bolster himself up ('comfort me in my disbelief'), Foch adduces a few citations, including the words of Marshal Bugeaud: 'Absolute principles are few, but they nevertheless obtain.'

But what comprises the first of these absolute principles, namely the principle of the economy of forces? The task of war is to overwhelm the enemy's living forces. This can be achieved only by means of a blow. For this blow a concentration of one's own forces is required. But before this blow can be dealt, it is necessary to discover the enemy's location, safeguard oneself against a sudden blow from his side, assure communications, and so on. This requires a disposition of corresponding detachments (reconnaissance, defense guards, etc.). The principle of economy of forces consists in assigning for auxiliary and preparatory tasks from among the basic detachments such forces—no more, no less—as are required by the very nature of these tasks; and at the same time, of assuring oneself at the decisive moment the possibility of bringing into play these auxiliary detachments in order to deal a concentrated blow. Foch explains that this result can be obtained only through the maneuverist offense of the basic army core as well as of the auxiliary detachments. The eternal principle of economy of forces is thus, according to Foch, characteristic only of maneuverist strategy. And it is hardly surprising that Foch permits into the holy of holies of military art only maneuverist offensive operations, holding that 'theories previously current among us are false.' Proceeding from maneuverist offense as the sole strategy, Foch predicts that the 'initial combat actions will prove decisive in the next war.' In harmony with this same view, Foch draws the 'conclusion that it [the next war] cannot be of long duration, and must be conducted with fierce energy and brought swiftly to its goal—otherwise it will be without results.'

In essence, it suffices to cite these conclusions in order for Foch's eternal principles to appear before us quite pathetically in the light of subsequent events. In the course of the last war the French army—after initial and costly attempts at offensives—went over to positional defense; the initial reverses did not at all predetermine the war's outcome as Foch had predicted; the war lasted four years; in essence, the war preserved throughout a positional character and was settled in the trenches; the first maneuverist period in the field served only to disclose the need of digging into the earth; the final period of field operations revealed only what had already been achieved in the trenches: the exhaustion of Germany's power of resistance.

This experience is of a certain value. If, according to Foch, the theories that dominated the French military school up to 1883 were false and the light of true principles began to dawn only toward the end of the last century, then a decade after his book was written it was already disclosed that the war had unfolded in complete contradiction to those predictions which Foch had deduced from eternal principles.

One might of course say that the error here is wholly on the side of Foch, who simply proved incapable of drawing the necessary conclusions from correct principles. But as a matter of fact, if the 'eternal' principle of economy of forces is stripped of Foch's incorrect conclusions, then not much remains of the principle itself. According to Foch's line of thought, which is here nourished in the main by the Napoleonic experience, it is necessary first of all to locate the enemy, safeguard oneself by bringing up necessary reconnaissance and defense units to the front, along the flanks and in the rear; and then, having outlined the basic direction of the blow, to subordinate all forces to a single overwhelming offensive action. Essentially, the bare principle of 'economy' of forces has nothing to do with all this. It all comes down to the pattern of the Napoleonic offensive maneuver in which all other considerations are subordinated to the moment of the concentrated blow.

The principle of economy of forces thus consists in an expedient distribution of forces between the basic and auxiliary units, all the while retaining the possibility of using all of them for the destruction of the enemy's living forces. However, the same Foch, basing himself on a famous conversation between Bonaparte and Moreau, gives another, more concrete and partial interpretation to the principle of economy of forces.

On returning from Egypt Bonaparte explained to Moreau how he had secured himself a superiority of forces in the face of numerical inferiority by first descending with all his forces upon a single flank, smashing it and utilizing the ensuing confusion in order to strike with all his forces at the other flank. Does this mean that from the 'theorem' (the expression is Foch's) of economy of forces is to be derived the principle of successive annihilation of the flanks? Obviously, no. We have here a specific case of a successful operation which is characterized by many most important elements: the number of troops, their armament, their respective mood, their disposition, the command, etc. In the concrete circumstances the problem was solved by Napoleon through one of several possible methods. Its successful outcome proves that Napoleon had the ability in the given instance of employing his forces; or, if you prefer, he used them economically; or he had applied the principle of 'economy of forces.' And nothing more.

But to interpret the principle of economy of forces in this way is only to give another name to the principle of expediency. This principle counsels us to act rationally, not to expend forces in vain. This smacks a little of—the 'principles' of Kuzma Prutkov. If I remain ignorant of military affairs as such then this principle will afford me nothing. With a mathematical law which states that the square of the hypotenuse is equal to the sum of the squares of the other two sides, I can confront every corresponding phenomenon and apply the theorem practically. But if all I know is the 'principle of economy of forces,' what can I do with it? It is only a mnemonic sign which can be of use only after one possesses all the corresponding practical knowledge and habits. Surprise, economy of forces, freedom of action, initiative, and so on and so forth—these are only mnemonic signs for someone learned in military affairs. 'Free masons' turned the signs of the mason's craft into freemasonic signs. Similarly, in military affairs a certain accumulated experience has a symbolic conditional denomination, that is all. There is nothing more.

Foch proves the absolute or eternal character of the principle of 'freedom of action' by tracing it back to Xenophon: 'Military art consists in an ability to retain freedom of action.' But what is the content of this freedom? First of all, freedom of initiative must be maintained as against the enemy, that is, he must not be given the opportunity to bind your will. In this general form the principle is quite incontestable. But it applies equally to fencing and to chess and generally to all forms of sport which involve two sides, and finally, to parliamentary and juridical debates. Foch later gives another interpretation to this same principle. Freedom of action is retained only by the commander-in-chief. All the other commanders are bound for they must act within the framework of his assignments. Consequently, their will is placed under the restraint not only of material circumstances, but also of formal prescriptions. But economy of forces, or common sense, or expediency—whichever you please—demands that the highest command not fix too narrow a framework for its subordinates. In other words, it is necessary to set a clearly defined goal, leaving to the subordinate command the maximum freedom of choosing and combining means for the realization of the set goal. In such a general form the principle is again incontestable. The difficulty in issuing orders, however, lies in finding that limit beyond which the definition of the desired goal already passes into inordinate supervision over the choice of means. The 'theorem' does not in and of itself provide any ready-made solution here. At best it serves only to remind the commander that he must find some solution to this problem.

But even apart from all this, it is quite clear that Foch gives an equivocal interpretation to the principle of freedom of action: On the one hand, it is that degree of initiative in battle which assures the necessary independence from the enemy's will; and on the other hand, it is a sufficiently wide freedom of maneuver for the lower command, within the limits of the goals and tasks fixed by the highest command.

Neither the former nor the latter interpretation can, however, be called a theorem, even in the broadest meaning of the word. In mathematics we understand by a theorem a correlation of variable magnitudes that holds good under all quantitative changes of these magnitudes. In other words, the equality is not disrupted by whichever arithmetical figures are substituted for the algebraic terms, designating the magnitudes. But what does the principle of economy of forces signify? Or the principle of freedom of action? Is this truly a theorem which permits, through a substitution of concrete magnitudes, of drawing correct practical conclusions? In no case. Any attempt actually to invest such a principle with 'absolute' meaning, that is, raise it to the degree of a theorem, results in vacuities like: It is necessary to use all forces expediently; it is necessary to retain initiative of action; it is necessary to issue expedient or realizable orders, and therefore exclude from them superfluous conditions, and so on. In such a form these are not at all military principles, *but axioms of all purposive human activity*.

But, in point of fact, among military theoreticians these and similar principles are given a far more concrete interpretation. That is, these principles are (either openly or surreptitiously) made to include regiments, corps and armies of a specific structure and armament, which operate on a basis of numerous statutes and regulations, summing up the experience of the past. In such a form there is nothing eternal about these eternal principles; and they in nowise resemble theorems, but are conditional denominations of certain methods, empirical habits, positive and negative experiences, etc., etc.

In the nature of things, all military theoreticians cannot escape from the following contradiction: In order to demonstrate the eternal character of the principles of military art they have to throw out the entire 'ballast' of living historical experience and reduce them to pleonasms, commonplaces, Euclidian postulates, logical axioms, etc. On the other hand, in order to demonstrate the importance of these principles in military affairs, they have to stuff these principles with the content of a specific epoch, a specific stage in the development of an army or in the development of military affairs; and thereby these principles are invested with the character of useful practical manuals for the memory.

These are not scientific generalizations but practical directives; not theorems, but statutes. They are not eternal, but transient. Their significance is all the greater, the less absolute they are, that is, the more they are filled with the concrete content of a given period of military affairs, its living peculiarities of organization, technique, and so on. They are not absolute but conditional. They constitute not a branch of science, but a practical manual of art.

Frederick the Great said: 'War is a science for those who are outstanding; an art for mediocrities; a trade for ignoramuses.' This statement is incorrect. There isn't and can't be a science of war, in the precise meaning of the word. There is the art of war. On the other hand, even a trade presupposes a schooling, and whoever has schooling is no ignoramus. It would be more correct to say that war is a skilled trade for the average individual and an art for an outstanding one. As regards an ignoramus, he is only the raw material of war; its cannon fodder, and not at all a skilled man.

The attempt to eternalize the Napoleonic principles proved, as we see, abortive. This was disclosed by the imperialist war. It could not have been otherwise, if only for the reason that the wars of the [French] revolution together with the Napoleonic wars that grew out of the former were distinguished by the colossal moral and political preponderance of the revolutionary French people and their army over the rest of Europe. The French took the offensive in the name of a new idea, closely bound up with the powerful interests of the popular masses. The opposing armies put up a half-hearted defense for the old system. But during the last imperialist war neither side was the bearer of a new principle embodied in a new revolutionary class. On both sides the war was imperialist in character, but, at the same time, the very existence of both sides, above all Germany and France, was equally threatened. There was no violent blow which would have immediately caused demoralization and dejection in the opposing camp; nor could such a blow have been struck in view of the great human and material strength of both camps who moved up all their forces and resources gradually.

For this reason the initial battles, in contrast to Foch's forecasts, did not at all predetermine the outcome of the war. For this very reason, offensives were shattered by counter-offensives and the armies, leaning more and more on their rear, dug into the earth. For this very same reason, the war lasted a long time—until the moral and material resources of one side were exhausted. The imperialist war thus went its course from beginning to end in violation of the 'eternal' maneuverist offensive principle proclaimed by Foch. This circumstance is underscored all the more by the fact that Foch turned out to be the victor, despite and against his own principles. The explanation for this is to be found in the fact that while Foch's principles were against him the English and American soldiers, and especially Anglo-American munitions, tanks and planes, were with him.

One may of course say that the principle of economy of forces remains valid for positional warfare as well. For in this case, too, an expedient distribution of forces between frontal detachments and the various categories of reserve is required. This is quite indisputable. But in such a general presentation, not even a trace remains of the scheme whereby forces are distributed for a concentrated offensive blow. The 'eternal' principle dissolves into a commonplace. In positional, defensive, offensive, as well as maneuverist wars it is necessary to have an expedient and economic distribution of forces depending upon the task at hand. It is quite self-evident that this 'eternal principle' applies to industry and commerce as much as to war. It is always necessary to utilize one's forces economically, that is, obtain maximum results from a minimum expenditure of energy. All human progress, and first of all, technology are based on this 'eternal' principle. Man began to use a stone axe, a club, etc., because he thus obtained the greatest results with the least expenditure of effort. Precisely for this same reason man went from the club to the spear and the sword. From them—to the gun and the bayonet, and later to the cannon, etc. For the very same reason, he now passes to the electric plow. The eternal principle of war thus comes down to a 'principle' which is the motor of all human development. As regards the concrete interpretation given by Foch to the principle of economy of forces, it proved to be an abortive attempt to give an absolute character to the Napoleonic offensive maneuver which is resolved by a concentrated blow.

And so, insofar as the principle of economy of forces is 'eternal,' it contains nothing military. And insofar as it is given a military interpretation, there is nothing eternal about it.

But why does all this talk about 'eternal' principles continue to persist? Because, as has already been pointed out, at the basis there is man. Human qualities undergo little change. Anatomical, physiological, psychological qualities alter slowly as compared to changes of social forms. The relation of man's hands and feet and the structure of his skull in our epoch are approximately the same as in the days of Aristotle. We know that Marx used to read Aristotle with delight. And were it possible to assume Aristotle's transfer to our epoch in order for him to read Marx's books, then in all likelihood Aristotle would have understood them excellently.

Man's anatomical and psycho-physical make-up is far more stable than social forms are. Corresponding to this there are two sides in military affairs: There is the individual side, which finds its expression in certain habits and methods, determined to a large measure by the biological nature of man, not eternal but stable; and there is the collective-historical side which depends on the social organization of man in war. But it is precisely this latter moment which decides the issue, because war begins when socially organized armed man enters into combat with another socially organized armed man. Otherwise we would have a fight—between animals.

ID, 1, b. Trotsky, Suvarov and Frunze'.* Having read the theses of Comrade Frunze, I skimmed through Suvorov's 'Science of Victory.' The designation, 'science' is of course incorrect; but Suvorov understood it in its most simplified form, that is, in the sense of that which must be assimilated.

* L. Trotsky, 'Our Current Basic Military Tasks', April 1 1922, *Military Writings*, pp. 89 ff.

Precisely in this sense the soldier, when made to run the gauntlet, was admonished: 'Here is science for you.' Under Suvorov's dictation Lieutenant-General Prevost de Lumian wrote down seven laws of war. Here they are:

1. *Act not otherwise than on the offensive.*

2. *When marching—speed is paramount; in attack—impetuosity, cold steel.*

3. *What we need is not methodism, but a correct military outlook.*

4. *All power to the commander-in-chief.*

5. *The enemy must be attacked and beaten in the field, that is, don't remain sitting in fortified regions but keep after the enemy.*

6. *Don't waste time on sieges. An open frontal assault is best of all.*

7. *Never divide forces for the sake of occupying points. If the enemy outflanks you, so much the better; the enemy is himself heading for defeat.*

What is this if not a proletarian doctrine?! This is almost word for word a strategy that 'flows from the class nature of the proletariat' and out of the civil war—only somewhat more succinctly and better stated! . . . Suvorov was of course in favor of the offensive. But he also said that we need not methodism but a correct military outlook . . . However, Suvorov, after all, led into battle a feudal army under the command of officer-nobles. It thus turns out that the principles of 'the offensive doctrine of the proletariat' coincide not only with the field statutes of bourgeois-imperialist France, but also with the military 'science' of the Suvorovist landlord-feudal Russia!

From this it does not at all follow that 'the laws of war are eternal,' as certain pedants say. Under discussion here are not at all laws in the scientific sense, but rather practical usages. Some of the simplest generalizations (as for example the advice—'attack, and so impetuously') apply to all forms of struggle between living creatures. Rule of thumb, speed, aggressiveness are necessary not only during clashes between two organized and armed forces, but also during a fist fight between two little boys and even when a hunting dog chases a rabbit. But if the seven Suvorovist commandments are not eternal laws of war, then it is even less possible to pass them off as the most modern principles of proletarian strategy.

Is there a difference between the Red Army and the army of Suvorov? There is. An enormous one. Incalculable. In the one case you have a feudal army, kept in darkness. Here you have an army that is revolutionary, and whose consciousness is growing. The aims are diametrically opposite. We are undermining everything that Suvorov defended. But this difference involves not a military doctrine but a class political world-outlook. In this little book, in his aphorisms, Suvorov also expounds a social world-outlook. Lacking it, Suvorov would not have been an army leader. Suvorov's entire psychologic art consisted in extracting the most out of the instrument represented by a feudal soldier. In his social doctrine Suvorov rested on two poles: gauntlets and 'God is with us.' In their place we have the Communist program and the Soviet constitution. . . .

So far as the questions of strategy are concerned, then here, as we see, the matter came down to this, that those who began by promising us a new proletarian doctrine, ended by copying out the rules of Suvorov, and made mistakes in copying.

*ID, 2. Savkin, 'Past Military Theorists'**

The very great general and political figure Napoleon Bonaparte (1769–1821) occupies a prominent place in the history of creation of bourgeois military art. As a general he developed in the turbulent years of the French bourgeois revolution of 1789–1794. Therefore, in evaluating the significance of Napoleon's theoretical and practical heritage it is necessary above all to consider the deciding role in changing the methods and forms of waging war which belongs to the French Revolution.

The revolution led to a rejection in strategy of methodical maneuver calculated to exhaust the enemy and to avoid decisive combat actions. Decisive military actions with the aim of defeating the enemy in an engagement became the basis. The new method of waging war rejected the linear distribution of forces for covering fortresses and important points and led

* Excerpts from V. Ye. Savkin, *Basic Principles of Operational Art and Tactics* (1972), pp. 17 f., 21, 24–7, 47.

to the delivery of powerful attacks by concentrated forces against enemy troops. In place of the old linear tactics came new shock tactics, based on a combination of bayonet and fire, columns and extended formation, which corresponded to the new, mass bourgeois army. The French bourgeois revolution produced a turnabout in the method of supplying troops. The old store system of supplying troops was eliminated and a new requisition system was introduced. In this manner mobility was achieved, which was unknown to the troops of their enemies, who were burdened with tents and all kinds of trains.

In explaining the reason for victories of the French bourgeois revolution, V. I. Lenin wrote: 'They refer constantly to heroic patriotism and wonders of military valor of the French in 1792–1793. But they forget about the material, historical-economic conditions which merely made these wonders possible.' The revolution created 'those material, economic conditions which saved France with 'wondrous' swiftness, having *regenerated and renewed* its economic basis.' This economic renewal of the country permitted creation of a previously unknown material base for organization of a massive bourgeois army. A large part was also played by the fact that 'the entire people,' write Lenin, 'and especially the masses, i.e., *the oppressed* classes, were gripped by a boundless revolutionary enthusiasm. All believed the war to be just and defensive, *and in fact* it was such. Revolutionary France defended itself against reactionary-monarchist Europe.'

Thus, the new bourgeois socio-economic and political relations became the basis for military successes of a new, massive army and for the elevation of Napoleon. Military science, created by the revolution, by military figures of the revolution, and by Napoleon, was the inevitable result of the new relationships born of the revolution. . . .

Henri Jomini (1779–1869), a major military theoretician and authority in the field of strategy in the first half of the 19th Century, devoted much attention to principles of military art in his works. He was by origin Swiss, and was a general in the French and later the Russian service.

Jomini's philosophical base is idealism. This predetermined his metaphysical views in questions of military affairs as well.

He proceeds from an assumption that principles of military art are eternal and unchangeable: 'The fundamental rules (of warfare),' he wrote, 'are unchangeable and are independent both of time and place.' Jomini did not see the development and change of military phenomena and their mutual ties. Jomini asserts that 'strategy was one and same both under Caesar and under Napoleon,' that eternal and immutable principles of strategy 'do not depend on the nature and attributes of weapons or the organization of troops.' . . .

At the turn of the 19th and 20th centuries, capitalism was developing into its highest and last stage—imperialism. Productive forces in the era of imperialism reached a very high level. This allowed creation of different forms of new combat equipment. In just the first 20 years of the 20th Century we saw created different models of automatic small arms, armored vehicles, combat aircraft, tanks, flame throwers, toxic substances, mortars, grenade launchers, antitank guns, etc. Mechanical means of transport and communications received great dissemination, and there began a process of motorization of armed forces. There was a sharp increase in the importance of economic and moral factors. New conditions and means of warmaking demanded fundamental changes in the field of military art.

Several works were published in the West at the end of the 19th and beginning of the 20th centuries which touched to one degree or another on the problem of principles of military art. Here, in spite of the development of a material basis of battles and operations during this period and the considerable changes in methods and forms of combat actions stemming from this, a majority of foreign military scholars lagged behind the science of their age and ignored the outstanding works of the founders of Marxism-Leninism on military questions and their only acceptable method of research. They remained on metaphysical and idealistic positions.

Rear Admiral Mahan (1840-1914) of the U.S. Navy, British Vice-Admiral Colomb (1831-1899), German General-Field Marshal A. Schlieffen (1833-1914), and other 'luminaries' of foreign military science considered the basis of military art to be 'eternal and unchanging principles of warmaking.' Colomb, for example, in the face of obvious facts stated: 'No one dared assert that railroads, the electric telegraph, breechloading guns and rifles changed the established principles of war-making on land.' Such frank statements embarrassed even dyed in the wool idealists and metaphysicians from among Colomb's contemporaries who held the same views.

Mahan nevertheless admitted, though with stipulations, certain changes in individual principles of tactics, but not in all. With regard to principles of strategy, they 'remain just as immovable as if on rock.'

As a result, the most well-known principles of military art of the ground armies formulated by writers and generals of the past were shifted by Mahan into a theory of war at sea. He diluted them with certain lessons of strategy of the sailing fleet. What came out was a misshapen hermaphrodite, and not naval strategy for a fleet which by that time was already fully powered by steam.

In the works of A. Schlieffen individual correct dialectical and even materialistic statements were oddly intertwined with clearly metaphysical and idealistic statements. Schlieffen correctly noted that 'war is only a means of politics' and that tactics change under the effects of new weapons. He said that it had already become unthinkable to attack enemy positions in columns similar to those of Napoleon, and it also was impossible to defeat an enemy using the fire of dense masses of riflemen. This did not hinder Schlieffen in declaring that, based on the 'eternal and unchangeable principles of military art,' there is an absolute idea of battle and an eternal, ideal prototype of war for which it is necessary to strive. 'Battle for destruction,' asserts Schlieffen, 'can even now be waged according to Hannibal's plan, drawn up in time immemorial.' . . .

Foch attempted to build military science from a position of subjective idealism, especially intuitivism and positivism. This inevitably led to a degeneration of military theory and to narrow practicalness. Foch's military system was not up to the demands for waging war of that time. The insolvency of his military system was a result primarily of the fallaciousness of his applied method and the narrowness of the base on which he built his conclusions. This base was some particular instance from the Napoleonic Wars or the Franco-Prussian War of 1870–1871 . . .

The main defect of Fuller's theory was an underestimation of the role of man and the significance of military science and an overestimation of the role of equipment in war. 'The cannons of war or weaponry, if only they meet the needs of the situation,' wrote Fuller, 'comprise 99 per cent of the victory. Strategy, command, control, bravery, discipline, supply, organization, and all moral and physical appurtenances of war are nothing in comparison with superiority in weapons; in the best instance they comprise 1 per cent.'

Fuller recognized the presence of principles of military art. He said: 'Similar to all other forms of human endeavor, war can be reduced to scientific foundations.' He made an appeal to reduce war 'to a system of knowledge based on specific principles.' Fuller's recognition of the development of military science is very noteworthy. Believing that military science 'is a living or dynamic science which must develop with the development of mankind,' he even fought for a revision of military science and at the very same time gave it an insignificant role—some fraction of a per cent—as is evident from the quote above. In addition, Fuller fell into an insoluble contradiction with his own view on the development of principles of military art, interpreting them as a manifestation in war of the universal, eternal, and unchanging law of nature—'the law of economy of force.'

IE. Mao, 'People Not Weapons'*

Hence the questions and the conclusions are as follows: 'Will China be subjugated? The answer is, No, she will not be subjugated, but will win final victory. Can China win quickly? The answer is, No, she cannot win quickly, and the war must be a protracted one. Are these conclusions correct? I think they are.

At this point, the exponents of national subjugation and of compromise will again rush in and say, 'To move from inferiority to parity China needs a military and economic power equal to Japan's, and to move from parity to superiority she will need a military and economic power greater than Japan's.

* Excerpts from Mao Tse-tung, 'On Protracted War', May 1938, *Selected Military Writings* (Peking, 1967), pp. 217 f., 225 f., 238 f.

But this is impossible, hence, the above conclusions are not correct.'

This is the so-called theory that 'weapons decide everything', which constitutes a mechanical approach to the question of war and a subjective and one-sided view. Our view is opposed to this; we see not only weapons but also people. Weapons are an important factor in war, but not the decisive factor; it is people, not things, that are decisive. The contest of strength is not only a contest of military and economic power, but also a contest of human power and morale. Military and economic power is necessarily wielded by people. If the great majority of the Chinese, of the Japanese and of the people of other countries are on the side of our War of Resistance against Japan, how can Japan's military and economic power, wielded as it is by a small minority through coercion, count as superiority? And if not, then does not China, though wielding relatively inferior military and economic power, become the superior? . . .

When we say we are opposed to a subjective approach to problems, we mean that we must oppose ideas which are not based upon or do not correspond to objective facts, because such ideas are fanciful and fallacious and will lead to failure if acted on. But whatever is done has to be done by human beings; protracted war and final victory will not come about without human action. For such action to be effective there must be people who derive ideas, principles or views from the objective facts, and put forward plans, directives, policies, strategies and tactics. Ideas, etc. are subjective, while deeds or actions are the subjective translated into the objective, but both represent the dynamic role peculiar to human beings. We term this kind of dynamic role 'man's conscious dynamic role', and it is a characteristic that distinguishes man from all other beings. All ideas based upon and corresponding to objective facts are correct ideas, and all deeds or actions based upon correct ideas are correct actions. We must give full scope to these ideas and actions, to this dynamic role. The anti-Japanese war is being waged to drive out imperialism and transform the old China into a new China; this can be achieved only when the whole Chinese people are mobilized and full scope is given to their conscious dynamic role in resisting

Japan. If we just sit by and take no action, only subjugation awaits us and there will be neither protracted war nor final victory. . . .

It is a human characteristic to exercise a conscious dynamic role. Man strongly displays this characteristic in war. True, victory or defeat in war is decided by the military, political, economic and geographical conditions on both sides, the nature of the war each side is waging and the international support each enjoys, but it is not decided by these alone; in themselves, all these provide only the possibility of victory or defeat but do not decide the issue. To decide the issue, subjective effort must be added, namely, the directing and waging of war, man's conscious dynamic role in war.

In seeking victory, those who direct a war cannot overstep the limitations imposed by the objective conditions; within these limitations, however, they can and must play a dynamic role in striving for victory. The stage of action for commanders in a war must be built upon objective possibilities, but on that stage they can direct the performance of many a drama, full of sound and colour, power and grandeur. Given the objective material foundations, the commanders in the anti-Japanese war should display their prowess and marshal all their forces to crush the national enemy, transform the present situation in which our country and society are suffering from aggression and oppression, and create a new China of freedom and equality; here is where our subjective faculties for directing war can and must be exercised. We do not want any of our commanders in the war to detach himself from the objective conditions and become a blundering hothead, but we decidedly want every commander to become a general who is both bold and sagacious. Our commanders should have not only the boldness to overwhelm the enemy but also the ability to remain masters of the situation throughout the changes and vicissitudes of the entire war. Swimming in the ocean of war, they must not flounder but make sure of reaching the opposite shore with measured strokes. Strategy and tactics, as the laws for directing war, constitute the art of swimming in the ocean of war. . . .

The thesis that incorrect subjective direction can change superiority and initiative into inferiority and passivity, and that correct subjective direction can effect a reverse change, becomes all the more convincing when we look at the record of defeats suffered by big and powerful armies and of victories won by small and weak armies. There are many such instances in Chinese and foreign history.

Among examples to be found abroad are most of Napoleon's campaigns and the civil war in the Soviet Union after the October Revolution. In all these instances, victory was won by small forces over big and by inferior over superior forces. In every case, the weaker force, pitting local superiority and initiative against the enemy's local inferiority and passivity, first inflicted one sharp defeat on the enemy and then turned on the rest of his forces and smashed them one by one, thus transforming the over-all situation into one of superiority and initiative. The reverse was the case with the enemy who originally had superiority and held the initiative; owing to subjective errors and internal contradictions, it sometimes happened that he completely lost an excellent or fairly good position in which he enjoyed superiority and initiative, and became a general without an army or a king without a kingdom. Thus it can be seen that although superiority or inferiority in the capacity to wage war is the objective basis determining initiative or passivity, it is not in itself actual initiative or passivity; it is only through a struggle, a contest of ability, that actual initiative or passivity can emerge. In the struggle, correct subjective direction can transform inferiority into superiority and passivity into initiative, and incorrect subjective direction can do the opposite. The fact that every ruling dynasty was defeated by revolutionary armies shows that mere superiority in certain respects does not guarantee the initiative, much less the final victory. The inferior side can wrest the initiative and victory from the superior side by securing certain conditions through active subjective endeavour in accordance with the actual circumstances.

IF. Byely, 'Dialectical Materialism and Its Application in Soviet Military Theory'*

Dialectical and historical materialism is one of the three component parts of Marxism and is, in fact, its philosophical basis. It combines philosophical materialism and materialist dialectics (dialectical materialism) and historical materialism. . . . It serves as the ideological and methodological basis for the development of science, including military science.

The most important feature of Marxist-Leninist philosophy, one that distinguishes it from all former and present philosophical systems, is its *capacity for unlimited creative development and improvement.* The possibilities for the development of Marxist-Leninist theory and its philosophical basis are just as unlimited and multifarious as human experience. Marxist-Leninist philosophy develops in indissoluble connection with practice, with the struggle for a revolutionary transformation of the world, for the ideological purity of revolutionary theory.

Laying the foundation for the new world outlook, Karl Marx wrote: 'The philosophers have only *interpreted* the world, in various ways; the point, however, is to change it.' This set a completely new task to philosophy—that of combining philosophy with practice, scientific communism with the activity of the working masses, with their struggle for the translation of revolutionary theory into practice.

With the victory of the Great October Socialist Revolution the link between theory and practice acquired qualitatively new features. When the proletariat won political power and the possibility emerged for realising the ideas of Marxism on a country-wide scale, Lenin wrote: '. . . *the historical moment has arrived when theory is being transformed into practice, vitalised by practice, corrected by practice, tested by practice'* (Author's emphasis.) . . .

The use of Marxist-Leninist philosophy for the solution of various problems is no simple matter. Historical experience shows that it is easier to learn definite propositions, formulas and principles of Marxist-Leninist philosophy than it is to

* Excerpts from B. Byely *et al., Marxism-Leninism on War and Army* (1972), pp. 378-87.

use them creatively for the solution of theoretical and practical tasks in the various fields of knowledge and in human activity. Lenin noted that such 'highly eminent Marxists' as Kautsky, Otto Bauer and others who had studied dialectics and taught it to others, turned out to be far from dialecticians when they applied them in life, in practice. To a great extent this applies also to Georgi Plekhanov, who did much to work out and disseminate Marxist philosophy, but was unable to apply it to the new historical conditions, to life, to the practice of the international communist movement.

Thus, it is one thing to know the propositions and formulas of Marxist–Leninist philosophy, and quite another to apply them in science and practice. The latter requires special skill. In turn, this skill presupposes a sustained, strictly consistent devotion to the Party, the adherence to a class point of view.

The elaboration of Soviet military doctrine, which has generalised the military experience in our epoch, the emergence and development of Soviet military science, are organically linked with Marxist–Leninist philosophy.

It would be illogical to demand of philosophy the solution of questions that are the subject-matter of military science. It would be equally wrong to attempt to resolve specific philosophical questions of military science without philosophy. This applies with special force when the question about the essence and content of war in general, and nuclear war in particular, is being analysed. Though recognising the dialectico-materialistic definition that war is the continuation of politics by violent means, some authors attempt to reduce war solely to the armed struggle, ignore its political content and belittle other forms of struggle during the war. In the heat of argument some even begin to prove that Lenin's proposition on war being the continuation of politics by violent means has become outmoded. Others approach this proposition dogmatically and refuse to see the changes that can take place in the essence and content of war. . . .

Key military problems are analysed with the help of Marxist–Leninist philosophy. It must be used in its entirety and it is inadmissible wilfully to apply some formulas, principles, laws and categories, while ignoring their relation to other principles, formulas or categories. . . .

The dialectical method of cognition is the way of achieving the truth, the way of the movement of thought, corresponding to the more general laws governing the development of the material world, to the nature of the objects, phenomena and processes of study. Its role in the development of all sciences, including Soviet military science, grows incessantly. The universal method of cognition and practical action is important because it is needed first and foremost by science itself, which develops rapidly while simultaneously going through a process of differentiation and integration. The growing importance of the universal method is conditioned also by the complexity of social practice in our highly dynamic and contradictory age. This is further determined by the internal laws governing the development of philosophy itself. Without reliance on dialectical materialism there can be no successful struggle against bourgeois ideology, against the ideology both of Right and 'Left' revisionism and nationalism. The universal method is growing in importance also because of the revolution in military affairs. The rapid change of some of the concepts and categories of military science, the change in the content of others, the new character of the interrelations between the various elements in military science, the limitations imposed on military practice, which is the motive force of the development of military science and a criterion of the correctness of its principles, all this assails military science with questions which cannot be resolved without a general philosophical method.

The immediate aim of science is *truth*, the final aim—*practice.* Every genuinely scientific truth is quite simple but the road leading to it is intricate. Dialectical materialism makes it possible to attain truth in the shortest way, to avoid many zigzags and deviations from objective truth. Dialectical materialism is an analogue of reality. That means that it is nothing but *the conscious use in cognition of the most general laws of the development of the objects, phenomena and processes.*

The demands of the dialectical method of cognition are an expression of the main laws and principles of Marxist-Leninist philosophy as applied to the scientific cognition of the material world. In this field philosophical laws and principles sometimes act as prerequisites, sometimes as essential standards of reasoning, as its rules. Let us examine the principal ones of them as applied to military affairs.

The principle of *objectivity* is the essential and initial principle of all scientific knowledge, it is based on the recognition of the objective nature of truth. As applied to military affairs this means that it is essential organically to combine a decisive, brave spirit with a comprehensive objective evaluation of the situation and the reliable provision of all the necessary means required by the troops during action. This forms the realistic Party approach, which is directly opposed to adventurism, so typical of the policy and strategy of the modern imperialist states. . . .

The strength of Soviet military science, its superiority over bourgeois military science, consists in the fact that it is guided by the Marxist-Leninist dialectical method and strives for the comprehensive study of all the principles and conditions for securing victory over the aggressor.

Several methodological demands evolve from the *principle of development.* The dialectico-materialist understanding of development, the general laws of movement, are a reliable general methodological basis for the solution of the fundamental problems of Soviet military science and practice. As applied to the process of cognition these laws act as important methodological demands.

The law of the mutual transformation of quantitative and qualitative changes obliges us to consider development in the military field in the unity of the quantitative and qualitative changes, in their mutual transitions. It enables us to understand the leap-like character of military development, the most profound expression of which is the modern revolution in the military field. Soviet military science, relying on dialectical materialism, correctly revealed the radical changes in military affairs, drew and continues to draw conclusions from them and to apply their results in the development of the Soviet Armed Forces, in the training and education of the personnel; it theoretically substantiates the application of new methods and forms of armed struggle in accordance with changes in military affairs.

The law of the unity and struggle of opposites, revealing the source of all development, gives rise to the general methodological demand which Lenin formulated as follows: 'The *reflection* of nature in man's thought must be understood not "lifelessly", not "abstractly", *not devoid of movement, NOT WITHOUT CONTRADICTIONS,* but in the eternal *PROCESS* of movement, the arising of contradictions and their solution.

War and military matters are distinguished by a particular contradictoriness. One cannot understand the socio-political content of every given war without first revealing the contradictions that have given rise to it. The armed struggle is a sharp contradiction, a duel of two opposing forces. Contradictions constantly emerge between weapons and military equipment, on the one hand, and the methods and forms of the armed struggle, on the other. The relations between defence and offensive, between the means of attack and the means of defence, between fire and movement, etc., are also contradictory.

Soviet military science is effective because it reveals the contradictions in military development consciously and opportunely and determines the ways and means for transcending them.

The methodological importance to military science of the *law of the negation of the negation,* which reveals the general trend of development, the relation of the old to the new in the development process, the spiral form of its ascendancy, consists in its demand for a critical, not a nihilistic, approach to the experience of the past, a critical and not nihilistic attitude towards bourgeois military science and equipment. It prevents military thought from stagnating and becoming rigid because it regards every stage in military development as a transition to a new, higher stage.

II. MARX AND ENGELS AS MILITARY THINKERS

Karl Marx (1818–83), the German economist and philosopher, and founder, along with Engels, of modern communism, was born in Trier, in the German Rhineland, the son of a lawyer. Best known as an economist—the first volume of his work *Das Kapital* appeared in 1867. His analysis formed the social and economic basis for the programmes of European social democracy, and contemporary Soviet and Chinese communism. In his later life, he believed his followers maintained and extended his views in too narrow and doctrinaire a spirit, and on one occasion protested 'I am not a Marxist.' Marx, like Engels, also wrote on military questions, but in this field he took second place to his collaborator.

Between 1851 and 1861, Marx was the London correspondent of the *New York Daily Tribune*. His decade of association with that paper was not only to provide him with a podium, but was an important source of financial support. Marx's link with the *Tribune* was Charles Anderson Dana, an American journalist whom he had met in Cologne in the revolutionary days of 1848. In 1851, Dana invited Marx to write for the *Tribune*, which, with its 200,000 readers, was the newspaper with the largest circulation in America. The editor-in-chief, Horace Greeley, was at this time a Fourierist, and therefore, like Dana and George Ripley, another editor of the *Tribune*, sympathetic to foreign socialists.

Marx's command of English was not up to the requirements of such journalism, and for the first year of his association with the *Tribune*, it was Engels who supplied the articles which were published under Marx's name. (In the following year, Engels translated Marx's German into an acceptable English, and in 1853, Marx began to write in English.) The Tribune paid £1 ($5) each for those articles it chose to print; in time, this fee was doubled and, for a few years, the paper even agreed to take two articles a week. The articles on the

Crimean War and the Indian Mutiny appeared in the *Tribune*. (Section IIA, B.)

With the coming of the Civil War, Dana quarreled with Greeley, who wished to make a compromise peace with the South, and very soon Marx found himself looking for a new outlet for his journalism. He turned to *Die Presse*, in Vienna, a daily with a circulation of about 30,000 (the largest in Austria), and appealing to the conservative middle-class of the metropolis. (*Die Presse* paid half the rate he had enjoyed during his last years on the *Tribune*.) Marx's chief pieces on the American Civil War appeared in this paper.

The articles in the *Tribune* and *Die Presse* all appeared under Marx's name, but it is clear from the Marx-Engels correspondence that some of them were almost entirely written by Engels. These articles on military matters are largely the work of Engels.

Marx and Engels were not merely neutral spectators of the Crimean War. For them, Russia was the chief enemy of all the causes they most valued. Not only was Russian power exerted, behind the scenes, to oppose all liberal and national movements in Europe, but the Tsar stood ready to intervene, if necessary, to support the forces of reaction. It had only been with the assistance of Russian troops, in 1848, that the Habsburgs were able to suppress the Hungarian Revolution. Marx and Engels were persuaded that it would first be necessary to crush Russian power if the social revolution to which they looked forward were to have a chance of early success. On the so-called Eastern Question which pitted Russia against Turkey throughout the nineteenth century, Marx and Engels were complete Turcophiles.

Engels' articles on the suppression of the Indian mutiny give further evidence of his technical competence as a military critic. His analysis of the siege of Delhi (section IIB) not only displays his understanding of the tactics of such a proceeding, but his professional doubts as to the strategic value of having undertaken the operation at all.

In the two articles which appeared in *Die Presse*, in 1862, on the American Civil War, Marx and Engels further revealed their considerable talents for military criticism. (Section IIG.) Indeed, they apparently understood the strategic considerations, on both sides of that struggle, rather better than many of the leading participants. Not only did they predict the failure of McClellan's 'anaconda' strategy, basing their view on a close knowledge of military history, they even outlined the strategy which was actually to be adopted to assure a Southern defeat.

From the beginning of the war, the sympathies of Marx and Engels were with the North, and they were disturbed that public opinion in Europe was equivocal, at best, and even in favour of the South. For the Socialist thinkers the war was not one for Southern self-determination or a free-trade policy, as it appeared to the London *Times*, or to the *Economist*, but one which the Northern democracy was waging against the retrograde slave-owners of the South.

Marx's old friend from Cologne, Charles A. Dana, along with his colleague on the *New York Daily Tribune*, George Ripley, had become the editors (in the years between 1858 and 1863) of the *New American Cyclopaedia*, published by the *Tribune*. Badly in need of money, Marx accepted Dana's invitation to write for the *Cyclopaedia*. Since Marx had supplied so much military correspondence to the *Tribune*, it seemed natural for Dana to commission him to prepare articles on military subjects for the encyclopaedia.

Marx, at times with Engels's help, prepared biographical articles on some of the French Marshals of the Napoleonic period and after, and a number of their Russian and German opponents. Engels, on the other hand, devoted himself to more technical pieces: on battles, on weapons, on the military branches (Artillery, Cavalry, Infantry, the Fleet), and the like. All display a highly professional competence. The most extensive articles, those in which Engels invested his greatest efforts, were the lengthy essays on 'Army' and 'Infantry'. Despite the view of them, in Communist Germany and Soviet Russia, as prime examples of proletarian military thinking, it is surprising how little of a specifically Marxist character they possess. (See Introduction.) This is less true of the essay on the 'proletarian' branch of the Infantry than that on the Army. (Section IIC.)

In his *Art of War*, Machiavelli had skilfully constructed the drama of the 'ideal' battle of his time. Clausewitz followed this example in his *On War*. In his article, 'Battle' for the *Cyclopaedia*, Engels described 'the average routine of a modern battle' against the background of the shapes of battles in the past. (Section IID.)

Between September 1860 and November 1861, Engels wrote ten articles for the *Volunteer Journal for Lancashire and Cheshire* in his role of a friendly critic of the Volunteer movement in England, set afoot by the fear of a French invasion which spread through the country in 1859. Engels was an earnest advocate of the Volunteers. Not only were they a defense against Bonapartism, but they clearly represented the kind of citizen-soldiers upon whom he must have based his hopes for a successful revolution. But the spirit that dominated his point of view was that of the professional soldier who wished to transform (as far as possible) raw groups of civilians into soldiers of the line, for Engels was convinced that there must be an immense gap between the volunteer and the professional. In these articles, Engels viewed with only the smallest sympathy the efforts of the bourgeois volunteers to elect officers, and with no sympathy at all the attempt of the landed magnates to assume the role of volunteer 'generals'. (Section IIE.)

Engels contributed five articles on the Austro-Prussian War of June and July 1866 to the *Manchester Guardian*. (Section IIH.) These pieces have special interest because Engels was at first convinced that Prussia would be defeated by the superior military techniques, capacities, and morale of the Austrian soldiers—this despite the fact that the Prussians were equipped with the breech-loading needle gun and the Austrians with the old-fashioned muzzle-loader. (See also Section IIF.) As the war progressed, the military critic concentrated his fire upon the Prussian disregard of the most elementary principles of strategy; this was certain to bring about their defeat. In time, however, Engels came to admire the fighting qualities—their 'tactical energy' making up for their 'strategic blunder'—of the Prussians, whose morale (inspired by hopes of German unification) was better than he had expected. And vital to Prussian victory, Engels now perceived, was the rapid-firing needle gun which he had discounted in his earlier articles.

Finally, we have Trotsky's highly favourable view of Engels's thoroughly pragmatic analysis of the Franco-Prussian war. If only, Trotsky mused in 1924, he had had these pieces in hand a couple of years earlier to display to the left-doctrinaire critics of his military programme. (Section IIJ.)

IIA. Marx and Engels, 'On the Crimean War'*

February 2 1854.—At last the long-pending question of Turkey appears to have reached a stage where diplomacy will not much longer be able to monopolize the ground for its ever-shifting, ever-cowardly, and ever-resultless movements. The French and the British fleets have entered the Black Sea in order to prevent the Russian navy from doing harm either to the Turkish fleet or the Turkish coast. The Czar Nicholas long since declared that such a step would be, for him, the signal for a declaration of war. Will he now stand it quietly?

It is not to be expected that the combined fleets will at once attack and destroy either the Russian squadron or the fortifications and navy-yards of Sebastopol. On the contrary, we may rest assured that the instructions which diplomacy has provided for the two admirals are so contrived as to evade, as much as possible, the chance of a collision. But naval and military movements once ordered, are subject not to the desires and plans of diplomacy, but to laws of their own which cannot be violated, without endangering the safety of the whole expedition. . . .

Until at least one of the German Powers is involved in a European war, the conflict can only rage in Turkey, on the Black Sea, and in the Baltic. The naval struggle must, during this period, be the most important. That the allied fleets can destroy Sebastopol and the Russian Black Sea fleet; that they can take and hold the Crimea, occupy Odessa, close the Sea of Azof, and let loose the mountaineers of the Caucasus, there is no doubt. With rapid and energetic action nothing is more easy. Supposing this to occupy the first month of active operations, another month might bring the steamers of the

* Excerpts from articles by K. Marx and F. Engels, *New York Daily Tribune*, Feb. 2, July 11, Aug. 17, 1854; Jan. 1, 22, 1855. [Articles republished in K. Marx and F. Engels, *The Russian Menace to Europe*, ed. P. W. Blackstock and B. F. Hoselitz (Glencoe, Ill.,: Free Press, 1952).]

combined fleets to the British Channel, leaving the sailing vessels to follow; for the Turkish fleet would then be capable of doing all the work which might be required in the Black Sea. To coal in the Channel and make other preparations, might take another fortnight; and then, united to the Atlantic and Channel fleets of France and Britain, they might appear before the end of May in the roads of Cronstadt in such a force as to ensure the success of an attack. The measures to be taken in the Baltic are as self-evident as those in the Black Sea. They consist in an alliance, at any price, with Sweden; an act of intimidation against Denmark, if necessary; an insurrection in Finland, which would break out upon landing a sufficient number of troops, and a guarantee that no peace would be concluded except upon the condition of this province being reunited to Sweden. The troops landed in Finland would menace Petersburg, while the fleets would bombard Cronstadt. This place is certainly very strong by its position. The channel of deep water leading up to the roads will hardly admit of two men-of-war abreast presenting their broadsides to the batteries which are established not only on the main island, but on smaller rocks, banks, and islands about it. A certain sacrifice, not only of men, but of ships, is unavoidable. But if this be taken into account in the very plan of the attack, if it be once resolved that such and such a ship must be sacrificed, and if the plan be carried out vigorously and unflinchingly, Cronstadt must fall. The masonry of its battlements cannot for any length of time withstand the concentrated fire of heavy Paixhan guns, that most destructive of all arms when employed against stone walls. Large screw-steamers, with a full complement of such guns amidships, would very soon produce an irresistible effect, though of course they would in the attempt risk their own existence. But what are three or four screw-ships of the line in comparison with Cronstadt, the key of the Russian Empire, whose possession would leave St. Petersburg without defence?

Without Odessa, Cronstadt, Riga, Sebastopol, with Finland emancipated, and a hostile army at the gates of the capital, with all her rivers and harbors closed up, what would Russia be? A giant without arms, without eyes, with no other recourse than trying to crush her opponents under the weight of her clumsy torso, thrown here and there at random, wherever a hostile battle-cry was heard. If the maritime powers of Europe should act thus resolutely and vigorously, then Prussia and Austria might so far be relieved from the control of Russia that they might even join the allies. For both the German Powers, if secure at home, would be ready to profit by the embarrassments of Russia. But it is not to be expected that Lord Aberdeen and M. Drouyn de l'Huys should attempt such energetic steps. The Powers that be are not for striking their blows *home*, and if a general war breaks out, the energy of the commanders will be shackled so as to render them innocuous. If nevertheless, decisive victories occur, care will be taken that it is by mere chance, and that their consequences are as harmless as possible for the enemy. . . .

But we must not forget that there is a sixth power in Europe, which at given moments asserts its supremacy over the whole of the five so-called 'great' Powers, and makes them tremble, every one of them. That power is the Revolution. Long silent and retired, it is now again called to action by the commercial crisis and by the scarcity of food. From Manchester to Rome, from Paris to Warsaw and Pesth, it is omnipresent, lifting up its head and awakening from its slumbers. Manifold are the symptoms of its returning life, everywhere visible in the agitation and disquietude which have seized the proletarian class. A signal only is wanted, and the sixth and greatest European power will come forward, in shining armor and sword in hand, like Minerva from the head of the Olympian. This signal the impending European war will give, and then all calculations as to the balance of power will be upset by the addition of a new element which, ever buoyant and youthful, will as much baffle the plans of the old European Powers, and their generals, as it did from 1792 to 1800.

July 11 1854.—Years of the dullest service, such as garrison duty and daily parade, and not youth, activity, and the study and acquirement of military science, have been the exclusive titles to the Czar's favour and to advancement. Thus the army is commanded on the average by old valetudinarians, or by ignorant corporals, who might manage a platoon, but have not brains and knowledge enough to direct the extensive and complicated movements of a campaign.

The same narrow-mindedness and presumption appear throughout the Czar's whole management of this Eastern Question. Every one can now see that he began the war in an unwise and inadequate manner. Indeed, his very first military demonstration was totally absurd and unequal to the purpose in hand. He ought to have known that Europe would not allow the destruction of Turkey, and should, therefore, either have kept quiet, biding his time, or have crossed the Pruth, not with between forty and fifty thousand men, as he did last year, when during the whole winter he had only one army corps in the Principalities, but should have pounced at once with his most powerful masses upon Turkey, reaching across the Balkans before the Turks could have gathered together their scattered forces, and before the Western Powers could have combined in their opposition and sent fleets of troops. To strike by surprise and terror ought to have been his aim, instead of engaging in such an imbecile manner his nation in a gigantic struggle. But Nicholas is growing old, and has all the faults of decrepit age. One of the reasons which prevented him from putting all his resources into action at once was that he feared the cost of such an effort. Now he will lose a hundred times as much money, and without results. Penny-wisdom in such an affair is no wisdom at all.

August 17 1857.—It would seem that whoever may have had any conservative leanings in Europe must lose them when he looks at this everlasting Eastern Question. There is all Europe, incapable, convicted for the last sixty years of incapability, to settle this puny little strife. There they are, France, England, Russia, going actually to war. They carry on their war for six months, and unless by mistake, or on a very shabby scale, they have not even come to blows. There they are, eighty or ninety thousand English and French soldiers, at Varna, commanded by old Wellington's late military secretary and by a Marshal of France (whose greatest exploits, it is true, were performed in London pawnshops)—there they are, the French doing nothing and the British helping them as fast as they can; and as they may think this sort of business not exactly honorable, the fleets are come up to Baltchik Roads to have a look at them and to see which of the two armies can enjoy the *dolce far niente* with the greater decorum. And, although the Allies have hitherto only been eating up the provisions upon which the Turkish army had calculated, idling away day after day at Varna, for the last two months, they are not yet fit for duty. They would have relieved Silistria if required by about the middle of May next year. The troops that have conquered Algeria had learned the theory and practice of war on one of the most difficult theatres in existence, the soldiers who fought the Sikhs on the sands of the Indus, and the Kaffirs in the thorny bush of South Africa, in countries far more savage than Bulgaria—there they are, helpless and useless, fit for nothing in a country which even exports corn!

But if the Allies are miserable in their performances, so are the Russians. They have had plenty of time to prepare. They have done whatever they could, for they knew from the beginning what resistance they would find. And yet, what have they been able to do? Nothing. They could not take a yard of contested ground from the Turks; they could not take Kalafat; they could not beat the Turks in one single engagement. And yet they are the same Russians who, under Muennich and Suvaroff, conquered the Black Sea coast from the Don to the Dniester. But Schilders is not Muennich, Paskevitch is not Suvaroff, and though the Russian soldier can bear flogging with the cane beyond all others, yet when it comes to habitual retreating he loses his steadiness as well as anybody else.

The fact is, that conservative Europe—the Europe of 'order, property, family, religion'—the Europe of monarchs, feudal lords, moneyed men, however they may be differently assorted in different countries—is once more exhibiting its extreme impotency. Europe may be rotten, but a war should have roused the sound elements, a war should have brought forth some latent energies; and assuredly there should be that much pluck among two hundred and fifty millions of men, that at least one decent struggle might be got up wherein both parties could reap some honor, such as force and spirit can carry off even from the field of battle. But no, not only is the England of the middle classes, the France of the Bonapartes, incapable of a decent, hearty, hard-fought war; but even Russia, the country of Europe least infected by infidel and unnerving civilization, cannot bring about anything of the kind. The Turks are fit for sudden starts of offensive action, and stubborn resistance on the defensive, but seem not to be fit for large combined maneuvers with great armies. Thus everything is reduced to a degree of impuissance and a reciprocal confession of weakness, which appears to be as reciprocally expected by all parties. With Governments such as they are at present, this Eastern war may be carried on for thirty years, and yet come to no conclusion.

January 1 1855.—If, in 1812, the Continental force launched against Russia was far weaker than that which she may perhaps see on her frontiers in April or May—if then England was her ally instead of her foe, Russia may console herself with the reflection that the more numerous the armies are which penetrate her interior, the more chance is there of their speedy destruction, and that, on the other hand, she has now three times the troops under arms which she had then.

Not that we think 'Holy Russia' unassailable. On the contrary, Austria and Prussia united are quite able, if merely military chances are taken into account, to force her to an ignominious peace. Any forty millions of men, concentrated upon a country of the size of Germany proper, will be able to cope successfully with the scattered sixty millions of Russian subjects. The strategy of an attack upon Russia from the west has been clearly enough defined by Napoleon, and had he not been forced by circumstances of a non-strategic nature to deviate from his plan, Russia's integrity would have been seriously menaced in 1812. That plan was to advance to the Dvina and the Dnieper, to organize a defensive position, both as to fortifications, depots, and communications, to take her fortresses on the Dvina, and to delay the march to Moscow until the spring of 1813. He was induced to abandon this plan, late in the season, from political reasons, from the outcry of his officers against winter quarters in Lithuania, and from a blind faith in his invincibility. He marched to Moscow, and the result is known. The disaster was immensely aggravated by the mal-administration of the French Commissariat, and by the want of warm clothing for the soldiers. Had these things been better attended to, Napoleon, on his retreat, might have found himself at Vilna at the head of an army twice in numbers that which Russia could oppose to him. His errors are before us; they are none of them of a nature irremediable; the fact of his penetrating to Moscow, the march of Charles XII to Poltava, prove that the country is accessible, though difficult of access; and as to maintaining a victorious army in its heart, that all depends upon the length of the line of operations from the Rhine to Eylau and Friedland, if we consider long lines of operations in their capacity of drawbacks upon the active force of an army, will be about equal to a line of operations from Brest-Litovsk (supposing the Polish fortresses to be taken in the first year) to Moscow. And in this supposition no account is taken of the circumstance that the immediate base of operations would have been advanced to Vitebsk, Mogilev, and Smolensk, without which preparatory act a march on Moscow would certainly be hazardous.

Russia is certainly thinly populated; but we must not forget that the central provinces—the very heart of Russian nationality and strength—have a population equal to that of central Europe. In Poland—that is, the five Governments constituting the Russian kingdom of Poland—the average is about the same. The most populous districts of Russia—Moscow, Tula, Riazan, Nijni-Novgorod, Kaluga, Yaroslavl, Smolensk, etc.—are the very heart of Great Russia, and form a compact body; they are continued, on the south, by the equally populous Little Russian provinces of Kiev, Poltava, Tehernigov, Voronezh, etc. There are, in all, twenty-nine provinces or governments, in which the population is quite half as dense as that of Germany. It is only the eastern and northern provinces, and the steppes of the south, where population is very thin; partly also the formerly Polish provinces of the west—Minsk, Mogilev, and Grodno—on account of extensive swamps between the (Polish) Bug and Dniester. But an advancing army, having in its rear the corn-producing plains of Poland, Volhynia, and Podolia, and in front, and for its theatre of operations, those of Central Russia, need not be afraid of its subsistence, if it manages the matter anything like well, and if it learns from the Russians themselves how to employ the means of transport of the country. As for a devastation of all resources by the retreating army, as in 1812, such a thing is only possible on one line of operations, and in its immediate vicinity; and if Napoleon had not, by his hurried advance from Smolensk, tied himself down to a very short time in which to complete his campaign, he would have found plenty of resources around him. But being in a hurry, he could not forage out the country at a short distance from his line of march, and his foraging parties, at that time, appear actually to have been afraid of penetrating far into the immense pine forests which separate village from village. An army which can detach strong cavalry parties to hunt up provisions, and the numerous carts and wagons of the country, can easily provide itself with everything necessary in the shape of food; and it is not likely that Moscow will burn down a second time. But even in that case, a retreat to Smolensk cannot be prevented, and there the army would find its well-prepared base of operation provided with every necessary.

January 22 1855.—It will be easily believed that the British army in the Crimea is in a state of complete disorganization—reduced to 'a mob of brave men,' as the London *Times* says—and that the soldiers may well welcome the Russian bullet which frees them from all their miseries.

But what is to be done? Why, unless you prefer waiting until half a dozen Acts of Parliament are, after due consideration by the Crown lawyers, discussed, amended, voted on, and enacted; until by this means the whole business connected with the army is concentrated in the hands of a real War Minister; until this new Minister, supposing him to be the right man, has organized the service of his office, and issued fresh regulations; in other words, unless you wait until the last vestige of the Crimean army has disappeared, there is only one remedy. This is the assumption by the General-in-Chief of the expedition, upon his own authority and his own responsibility, of that dictatorship over all the conflicting and contending departments of the military administration which every other General-in-Chief possesses, and without which he cannot bring the enterprise to any end but ruin. That would soon make matters smooth; but where is the British general who would be prepared to act in this Roman manner, and on his trial defend himself, like the Roman, with the words, 'Yes, I plead guilty to having saved my country'?

Finally we must inquire who is the founder and preserver of this beautiful system of administration. Nobody but the old Duke of Wellington. He stuck to every detail of it as if he was personally interested in making it as difficult as possible for his successors to rival him in war-like glory. Wellington, a man of eminent common sense, but of no genius whatever, was the more sensible of his own deficiencies in this respect from being the contemporary and opponent of the eminent genius of Napoleon. Wellington, therefore, was full of envy of the success of others. His meanness in disparaging the merits of his auxiliaries and allies is well known; he never forgave Blücher for saving him at Waterloo. Wellington knew full well that had not his brother been minister during the Spanish War he never could have brought it to a successful close. Was Wellington afraid that future exploits would place him in the shade? And did he therefore preserve to its full extent this machinery so well adapted to fetter generals and to ruin armies?

IIB. Marx and Engels, 'Capture of Delhi'*

If we compare Delhi with Sevastopol, we of course agree that the sepoys were no Russians; that none of their sallies against the British cantonment was anything like Inkermann; that there was no Todtleben in Delhi, and that the sepoys, bravely as every individual man and company fought in most instances, were utterly without leadership, not only for brigades and divisions, but almost for battalions; that their cohesion did not therefore extend beyond the companies; that they entirely lacked the scientific element without which an army is nowadays helpless, and the defence of a town utterly hopeless. Still, the disproportion of numbers and means of action, the superiority of the sepoys over the Europeans in withstanding the climate, the extreme weakness to which the force before Delhi was at times reduced, make up for many of these differences,

* Excerpts from K. Marx and F. Engels, *New York Daily Tribune,* Dec. 5 1857. [Article republished in S. Avineri, ed., *Karl Marx on Colonialism and Modernization* (New York: Doubleday, 1968).]

and render a fair parallel between the two sieges (to call these operations sieges) possible. Again we do not consider the storming of Delhi as an act of uncommon or extra-heroic bravery, although as in every battle individual acts of high spirit no doubt occurred on either side, but we maintain that the Anglo-Indian army before Delhi has shown more perseverance, force of character, judgement and skill, than the English army when on its trial between Sevastopol and Balaklava. The latter, after Inkermann, was ready and willing to re-embark, and no doubt would have done so if it had not been for the French. The former, when the season of the year, the deadly maladies consequent upon it, the interruption of the communications, the absence of all chance of speedy reinforcements, the condition of all Upper India, invited a withdrawal, did indeed consider the advisability of this step, but for all that, held out at its post.

When the insurrection was at its highest point, a movable column in Upper India was the first thing required. There were only two forces that could be thus employed—the small force of Havelock, which soon proved inadequate, and the force before Delhi. That it was, under these circumstances, a military mistake to stay before Delhi, consuming the available strength in useless fights with an unassailable enemy; that the army in motion would have been worth four times its value when at rest; that the clearing of Upper India, with the exception of Delhi, the re-establishing of the communications, the crushing of every attempt of the insurgents to concentrate a force, would have been obtained, and with it the fall of Delhi, as a natural and easy consequence, are indisuptable facts. But political reasons commanded that the camp before Delhi should not be raised. It is the wiseacres at headquarters who sent the army to Delhi that should be blamed—not the perseverance of the army in holding out when once there. At the same time we must not omit to state that the effect of the rainy season on this army was far milder than was to be anticipated, and that with anything like an average amount of the sickness consequent upon active operations at such a period, the withdrawal or the dissolution of the army would have been unavoidable. The dangerous position of the army lasted till the end of August. The reinforcements began to come in, while dissensions continued to weaken the rebel camp. In the beginning of September the siege-train arrived, and the defensive position was changed into an offensive one. On the 7th of September the first battery opened its fire, and on the evening of the 13th two practicable breaches were opened. Let us now examine what took place during this interval.

The English had strengthened the defences of Delhi so far that they could resist a siege by an Asiatic army. According to our modern notions, Delhi was scarcely to be called a fortress, but merely a place secured against the forcible assault of a field force. Its masonry wall, 16 feet high and 12 feet thick, crowned by a parapet of 3 feet thickness and 8 feet height, offered 6 feet of masonry besides the parapet, uncovered by the glacis and exposed to the direct fire of the attack. The narrowness of this masonry rampart put it out of the question to place cannon anywhere, except in the bastions and Martello towers. These latter flanked the curtain but very imperfectly, and a masonry parapet of three feet thickness being easily battered down by siege guns (field pieces could do it), to silence the fire of the defence, and particularly the guns flanking the ditch, was very easy. Between wall and ditch there was a wide berm or level road, facilitating the formation of a practicable breach, and the ditch, under these circumstances, instead of being a *coupegorge* for any force that got entangled in it, became a resting place to re-form those columns that had got into disorder while advancing on the glacis.

To advance against such a place, with regular trenches, according to the rules of sieges, would have been insane, even if the first condition had not been wanting, viz., a force sufficient to invest the place on all sides. The state of the defences, the disorganization and sinking spirit of the defenders, would have rendered every other mode of attack than the one pursued an absolute fault. This mode is very well known to military men under the name of the forcible attack (*ataque de vive force*). The defences, being such only as to render an open attack impossible without heavy guns, are dealt with summarily by the artillery; the interior of the place is all the while shelled, and as soon as the breaches are practicable the troops advance to the assault.

The front under attack was the northern one, directly

opposite to the English camp. This front is composed of two curtains and three bastions, forming a slightly re-entering angle at the central (the Cashmere) bastion. The eastern position, from the Cashmere to the Water bastion, is the shorter one, and projects a little in front of the Western position, between the Cashmere and the Moree bastions. The ground in front of the Cashmere and Water bastions was covered with low jungle, gardens, houses, etc., which had not been levelled down by the sepoys, and afforded shelter to the attack. (This circumstance explains how it was possible that the English could so often follow the sepoys under the very guns of the place, which was at that time considered extremely heroic, but was in fact a matter of little danger so long as they had this cover.) Besides, at about 400 or 500 yards from this front, a deep ravine ran in the same direction as the wall, so as to form a natural parallel for the attack. The river, besides, giving a capital basis to the English left, the slight salient formed by the Cashmere and Water bastions was selected very properly as the main point of attack. The western curtain and bastions were simultaneously subjected to a simulated attack, and this manœuvre succeeded so well that the main force of the sepoys was directed against it. They assembled a strong body in the suburbs outside the Cabul gate, so as to menace the English right. This manœuvre would have been perfectly correct and very effective, if the western curtain between the Moree and Cashmere bastions had been the most in danger. The flanking position of the sepoys would have been capital as a means of active defence, every column of assault being at once taken in flank by a movement of this force in advance. But the effect of this position could not reach as far eastward as the curtain between the Cashmere and Water bastions; and thus its occupation drew away the best part of the defending force from the decisive point.

The selection of the places for the batteries, their construction and arming, and the way in which they were served, deserve the greatest praise. The English had about 50 guns and mortars, concentrated in powerful batteries, behind good solid parapets. The sepoys had, according to official statements, 55 guns on the attacked front, but scattered over small bastions and Martello towers, incapable of concentrated action, and scarcely sheltered by the miserable three feet parapet. No doubt a couple of hours must have sufficed to silence the fire of the defence, and then there remained little to be done.

On the 8th, No. 1 battery, 10 guns, opened fire at 700 yards from the wall. During the following night the ravine aforesaid was worked out into a sort of trench. On the 9th, the broken ground and houses in front of this ravine were seized without resistance; and on the 10th, No. 2 battery, 8 guns, was unmasked. This latter was 500 or 600 yards from the wall. On the 11th, No. 3 battery, built very boldly and cleverly at 200 yards from the Water bastion in some broken ground, opened fire with six guns, while ten heavy mortars shelled the town. On the evening of the 13th, the breaches—one in the curtain adjoining the right flank of the Cashmere bastion, and the other in the left face and flank of the Water bastion—were reported practicable for escalade, and the assault was ordered. The sepoys on the 11th had made a counter-approach on the glacis between the two menaced bastions, and threw out a trench for skirmishers about three hundred and fifty yards in front of the English batteries. They also advanced from this position outside the Cabul gate to flank attacks. But these attempts at active defence were carried out without unity, connection or spirit, and led to no result.

At daylight on the 14th, five British columns advanced to the attack. One, on the right, to occupy the force outside the Cabul gate and attack, in case of success, the Lahore gate. One against each breach, one against the Cashmere gate, which was to be blown up, and one to act as a reserve. With the exception of the first, all these columns were successful. The breaches were but slightly defended, but the resistance in the houses near the wall was very obstinate. The heroism of an officer and three sergeants of the Engineers (for here there *was* heroism) succeeded in blowing open the Cashmere gate, and thus this column entered also. By evening the whole northern front was in the possession of the English. Here Gen. Wilson, however, stopped. The indiscriminate assault was arrested, guns brought up and directed against every strong position in the town. With the exception of the storming of the magazine, there seems to have been very little actual fighting. The insurgents were dispiritied and left the town in masses. Wilson advanced cautiously into the town, found scarcely any resistance after the 17th, and occupied it completely on the 20th.

Our opinion on the conduct of the attack has been stated. As to the defence—the attempt at offensive counter-movements the flanking position at the Cabul gate, the counter-approaches, the rifle-pits, all show that some notions of scientific warfare had penetrated among the sepoys; but either they were not clear enough, or not powerful enough, to be carried out with any effect. Whether they originated with Indians, or with some of the Euorpeans that are with them, is of course difficult to decide; but one thing is certain: that these attempts, though imperfect in execution, bear a close resemblance in the groundwork to the active defence of Sevastopol, and that their execution looks as if a correct plan had been made for the sepoys by some European officer, but that they had not been able to understand the idea fully, or that disorganization and want of command turned practical projects into weak and powerless attempts.

IIC. Engels, 'Infantry'*

Such was the army and such were the tactics which Frederic II of Prussia found at his disposal on his accession. There appeared to be very little chance for a man of genius to improve upon this system, unless he broke through it, and that Frederic, in his position and with the material he had for soldiers, could not do. Still he contrived to organize his mode of attack and his army so that he could, with the resources of a kingdom less than Sardinia now is, and with scanty pecuniary support from England, carry on a war against almost all Europe. The mystery may be easily explained. Hitherto the battles of the 18th century had been parallel battles, both armies being deployed on lines parallel to each other, struggling in a plain, fair, stand-up fight, without any strategems or devices of art; the only advantage accruing to the stronger party being that his wings overlapped those of his opponent. Frederic applied to the line order of battle the system of oblique attack invented

* Article, 'Infantry' (F. Engels), in *New American Cyclopaedia* (1858).

by Epaminondas. He chose one wing of the enemy for the first attack, and brought against this one of his wings, overlapping that of the enemy, and part of his centre, at the same time keeping back the rest of his army. Thus not only had he the advantage of outflanking the enemy, but also of crushing by superior forces the troops exposed to his attack. The other troops of the enemy could not come to the assistance of those attacked; for not only were they tied to their places in the line, but as the attack on the one wing proved successful the remainder of the army entered into line and engaged the hostile centre in front, while the original attacking wing fell upon its flank after disposing of the wing. This was indeed the only imaginable method by which it was possible, while maintaining the system of lines, to bring a superior force upon any one part of the enemy's line of battle. Every thing, then, depended upon the formation of the attacking wing; and as far as the rigidity of the order of battle admitted of it, Frederic always stengthened it. He very often placed in front of the first line of infantry of the attacking wing an advanced line formed of his grenadiers or élite troops, so as to insure success as much as possible at the first onset. The second means which Frederic took to improve his army was the reorganization of his cavalry. The teachings of Gustavus Adolphus had been forgotten; cavalry, instead of relying on the sword and the impetuosity of the charge, with rare exceptions had returned to fighting with the pistol and the carbine. The wars in the beginning of the 18th century had thus not been rich in successful charges of horsemen; the Prussian cavalry was especially neglected. But Frederic returned to the old plan of charging sword in hand and at full gallop, and formed a cavalry unequalled in history; and to this cavalry he owed a very great part of his successes. When his army became the model of Europe, Frederic, in order to blind the military men of other nations, began to complicate to an astonishing degree the system of tactical evolutions, all of them unfit for actual war, and intended only to hide the simplicity of the means which had procured him victory. He succeeded so well in this that nobody was more blinded than his own subordinates, who actually believed that these complex methods of forming line were the real essence of his tactics; and thus Frederic, beside laying the foundation for that pedantry and martinetism which have since distinguished the Prussians, actually prepared them for the unparalleled disgrace of Jena and Auerstädt.—Beside the infantry of the line which we have so far described, and which always fought in closed ranks, there was a certain class of light infantry, but this did not appear in great battles. Its task was the war of partisans; for this the Austrian Croats were admirable adapted, while for every other purpose they were useless. Upon the model of these half savages from the military frontier against Turkey, the other European states formed their light infantry. But skirmishing in great battles, such as was practised by the light infantry of antiquity and of the middle ages, even up to the 17th century, had completely disappeared. The Prussians alone, and after them the Austrians, formed a battalion or two of riflemen, composed of gamekeepers and forest guards, all dead shots, who in battle were distributed over the whole front and fired at officers; but they were so few that they scarcely counted. The resuscitation of skirmishing is the product of the American war of independence. While the soldiers of European armies, held together by compulsion and severe treatment, could not be trusted to fight in extended order, in America they had to contend with a population which, untrained to the regular drill of line soldiers, were good shots and well acquainted with the rifle. The nature of the ground favored them; instead of attempting manœuvres of which at first they were incapable, they unconsciously fell into skirmishing. Thus, the engagement of Lexington and Concord marks an epoch in the history of infantry. VII. THE INFANTRY OF THE FRENCH REVOLUTION AND OF THE 19TH CENTURY. When the European coalition invaded revolutionary France, the French were in a similar position to that of the Americans a short time before, except that they had not the same advantages of ground. In order to fight the numerous armies, invading or threatening to invade the country, upon the old line principle, they would have required well drilled men, and these were scarce, while undrilled volunteers were plentiful. As far as time allowed, they were exercised in the elementary evolutions of linear tactics; but as soon as they got under fire, the battalions deployed in line dissolved themselves, unconsciously, into thick swarms of skirmishers, seeking protection against fire from all accidents of ground, while the second line formed a kind of reserve which often enough was involved in the fight from the very beginning of the engagement. The French armies, moreover, were very differently organized from those opposed to them. They were formed, not into an unbending monotonous line of battalions, but into army divisions, each of which was composed of artillery, cavalry, and infantry. The great fact was all at once rediscovered that it matters not whether a battalion fights in its 'correct' place in the order of battle, so that it advances into line when ordered, and fights well. The French government being poor, tents and the immense baggage of the 18th century were done away with; bivouacking was invented, and the comforts of the officers, which in other armies formed a large portion of the impediments, were reduced to what they could carry on their backs. The army, instead of being fed from magazines, had to depend upon requisitions on the country passed through. Thus the French attained a mobility and a facility of forming order of battle quite unknown to their enemies. If beaten, they were out of the reach of pursuit in a few hours; if advancing, they could appear on unexpected points, on the flanks of the enemy, before he got notice. This mobility, and the jealousy among themselves of the chiefs of the coalition, gave them breathing time to drill their volunteers, and to elaborate the new tactical system which was rising among them. From the year 1795 we find this new system taking the definite form of a combination of skirmishers and close columns. The formation in line was subsequently added, though not for a whole army as hitherto, but for single battalions only, which deployed in line whenever an opportunity appeared to require it. It is evident that this latter manœuvre, requiring more steadiness of drill, was the last to be resumed by the irregular bands of the French revolution. Three battalions formed a demi-brigade, 6 a brigade; 2 or 3 brigades of infantry a division, to which were added 2 batteries of artillery and some cavalry; several such divisions formed an army. Whenever a division met the enemy, the skirmishers of its advanced guard established themselves in a defensive position, the advanced guard forming their reserve until the division came up. The brigades then formed upon two lines and a reserve, but every battalion in column, and with no stated intervals; for the protection of rents in the order of battle there was the cavalry and the reserve. The line of battle was no longer necessarily a straight and uninterrupted one; it might be bent in all directions, as the ground required, for now there was no longer a selection of naked level plains for battle fields; on the contrary, the French preferred broken ground, and their skirmishers, forming a chain in front of the whole line of battle, threw themselves into every village, farm yard, or copse that they could get hold of. If the battalions of the first line deployed, they generally all turned now soon skirmishers; those of the second line always remained in column, and generally charged in this formation against the thin lines of the enemy with great success. Thus, the tactical formation of a French army for battle gradually came to consist of two lines, each formed of battalions in close column placed *en èchiquier*, with skirmishers before the front, and a compact reserve in the rear. It was at this stage of development that Napoleon found the tactics of the French revolution. As soon as his accession to political power allowed him to do so, he began to develop the system still further. He concentrated his army in the camp of Boulogne, and there gave them a regular course of drill. He especially practised them in the formation of compact reserve masses on a small space of ground, and in the quick deployment of these masses for entering into line. He formed 2 or 3 divisions into one army corps so as to simplify the command. He invented and brought to its highest perfection the new marching order, which consists in spreading the troops over so great an extent of ground that they can subsist on the stores it contains, still keeping so well together that they can be united on any given point before the part which is attacked can be crushed by the enemy. From the campaign of 1809, Napoleon began to invent new tactical formations, such as deep columns of entire brigades and divisions, which however signally failed and were never again revived. After 1813 this new French system became the common property of all nations on the continent of Europe. The old line system, and the system of recruiting mercenaries, had both been abandoned. Everywhere the liability of every citizen to military service was acknowledged, and everywhere the new tactics were introduced. In Prussia and Switzerland every one had actually to serve; in the other states a conscription was introduced, the young men drawing lots to determine who should serve; everywhere reserve systems were introduced, by dismissing a portion of the men, when drilled, to their homes, so as to have a large number of drilled men at disposal in case of war, with little expense in peace.—Since that time several changes have occurred in the armament and organization of infantry, produced partly by the progress of the manufacture of small arms, partly by the collision of French infantry with the Arabs of Algeria. The Germans, always fond of the rifle, had increased their battalions of light riflemen; the French, driven by the necessity of having in Algeria an arm of greater range, at last in 1840 formed a battalion of riflemen armed with an improved rifle of great precision and range. These men, drilled to perform all their evolutions and even long marches in a kind of trot (*pas gymnastique*), soon proved themselves of such efficiency that new battalions were formed. In this manner a new light infantry was created, not from sporting shots and gamekeepers, but from the strongest and most agile men; precision of fire and long range were combined with agility and endurance, and a force was formed which, as far as it went, was certainly superior to any other infantry in existence. At the same time, the *pas gymnastique* was introduced into the infantry of the line, and what even Napoleon would have considered the height of folly, running, is now practised in every army as an essential part of infantry drill. The success of the new rifle of the French riflemen (Delvigne-Pontchara) soon produced new improvements. The conical bullet was introduced for rifled arms. New means were invented by Minié, Lorenz, and Wilkinson, to make the bullet glide down easily into the bore, and still to expand it, when once down, so as to fill up the grooves with its lead, and thus to give it the lateral rotation and force on which the effect of the rifle depends; on the other hand, Dreyse invented the needle gun, to be loaded at the breech, and not requiring a separate priming. All these rifles were capable of hitting at 1,000 yards, and quite as easily loaded as a common smooth-bore musket. Then the idea arose of arming the whole of the infantry with such rifles. England was the first to carry out this idea; Prussia, which had prepared for this step long before, followed; then Austria and the smaller German states; at last France. Russia, and the Italian and Scandinavian states, are still behind. This new armament has completely changed the aspect of warfare, but not in the way expected by tactical theorists, and for a very simple mathematical reason. It can be easily proved, by constructing the flight of these bullets, that an error of 20 or 30 yards in the estimation of the distance of the object will destroy all chance of hitting beyond 300 or 350 yards. Now, while on the practice ground the distances are known, on the battle field they are not, and they change every moment. Infantry posted in a defensive position, and having had time to pace off the distances of the most conspicuous objects before the front, will thus have an immense advantage, at from 1,000 to 300 yards, over an attacking force. This can only be obviated by advancing rapidly and without firing, at full trot, to some 300 yards when the fire of the two parties will be equally effective. At this distance firing will become so murderous between two well posted lines of skirmishers, and so many bullets will hit the pickets and reserves, that a plucky infantry can do no better than seize the first opportunity to make a rush at the enemy, giving a volley at 40 or 50 yards. These rules, first proved theoretically by the Prussian Major Trotha, have been practically tried by the French in their late war against the Austrians, and with success. They will, therefore, form part and parcel of modern infantry tactics, especially if they prove to be of equally good effect when tried against such a rapidly loading arm as the Prussian needle gun. The arming of all infantry with one and the same rifle gun will tend to do away with the distinctions, still existing, of light and line infantry, by forming an infantry capable of any service. In this will evidently consist the next improvement of this arm.

IID. Engels, 'Battle'*

BATTLE. The encounter of two hostile bodies of troops is called a battle, when these bodies form the main armies of

* Article, 'Battle' (F. Engels), in *New American Cyclopaedia* (1858).

either party, or at least, are acting independently on their own separate seat of war. Before the introduction of gunpowder, all battles were decided by actual hand-to-hand fight. With the Greeks and Macedonians, the charge of the close phalanx bristling with spears, followed up by a short engagement with the sword, brought about the decision. With the Romans, the attack of the legion disposed in three lines, admitted of a renewal of the charge by the second line, and of decisive manœuvring with the third. The Roman line advanced up to within 10 or 15 yards of the enemy, darted their *pila*, very heavy javelins, into him, and then closed sword in hand. If the first line was checked, the second advanced through the intervals of the first, and if still the resistance was not overcome, the third line, or reserve, broke in upon the enemy's centre, or fell upon one of his wings. During the middle ages, charges of steel-clad cavalry of the knights had to decide general actions, until the introduction of artillery and small fire-arms restored the preponderance of infantry. From that time the superior number and construction of fire-arms with an army was the chief element in battle, until, in the 18th century, the whole of the armies of Europe had provided their infantry with muskets and were about on a par as to the quality of their fire-arms. It was then the number of shots fired in a given time, with average precision which became the decisive element. The infantry was drawn up in long lines, three deep; it was drilled with the minutest care, to insure steadiness and rapid firing, up to 5 times in a minute; the long lines advanced slowly against each other, firing all the while, and supported by artillery firing grape; finally, the losses incurred by one party caused the troops to waver, and this moment was seized by the other party for an advance with the bayonet, which generally proved decisive. If one of the two armies, before the beginning of the battle, had already taken up its position, the other attempted generally to attack it under an acute angle, so as to outflank, and there to envelope, one of his wings; that wing, and the nearest portion of the centre, were thus thrown into disorder by superior forces, and crowded together in deep masses, upon which the attacking party played with his heavy artillery. This was the favorite manœuvre of Frederic the Great, especially successful at Leuthen. Sometimes, too, the cavalry was let loose upon the wavering infantry of the enemy, and in many instances with signal success; but upon the whole, the quick fire of the infantry lines gave the decision—and this fire was so effective, that it has rendered the battles of this period the bloodiest of modern times. Frederic the Great lost, at Kolin 12,000 men out of 18,000, and at Kunersdorf, 17,000 out of 30,000, while in the bloodiest battle of all Napoleon's campaigns, at Borodino, the Russians lost not quite one-half of their troops in killed and wounded. The French revolution and Napoleon completely changed the aspect of battles. The army was organized in divisions of about 10,000 men, infantry, cavalry, and artillery mixed; it fought no longer in line exclusively, but in column and in skirmishing order also. In this formation it was no longer necessary to select open plains alone for battlefields; woods, villages, farm-yards, any intersected ground was rather welcome than otherwise. Since this new formation has been adopted by all armies, a battle has become a very different thing from what it was in the 18th century. Then, although the army was generally disposed in three lines, one attack, or at most two or three attacks, in rapid succession, decided its fate; now, the engagement may last a whole day, and even two or three days, attacks, counter-attacks, and manoeuvres succeeding each other, with varying success, all the time through. A battle, at the present day, is generally engaged by the advanced guard of the attacking party sending skirmishers out with their supports. As soon as they find serious resistance, which generally happens at some ground favorable for defence, the light artillery, covered by skirmishers and small bodies of cavalry, advances, and the main body of the advanced guard takes position. A cannonade generally follows, and a deal of ammunition is wasted, in order to facilitate reconnoitring, and to induce the enemy to show his strength. In the mean time, division after division arrives, and is shown into its fighting position, according to the knowledge so far obtained of the measures of the enemy. On the points favoring an attack, skirmishers are sent forward, and supported where necessary by lines and artillery; flank attacks are prepared, troops are concentrated for the attack of important posts in front of the main position of the enemy, who makes his arrangements accordingly. Some manœuvring takes place, in order to threaten defensive positions, or to menace a threatening attack with a counter-charge. Gradually the army draws nearer to the enemy, the points of attack are finally fixed, and the masses advance from the covered positions they hitherto occupied. The fire of infantry in line, and of artillery, now prevails, directed upon the points to be attacked; the advance of the troops destined for the charge follows, a cavalry charge on a small scale occasionally intervening. The struggle for important posts has now set in; they are taken and retaken, fresh troops being sent forward in turns by either party. The intervals between such posts now become the battle-field for deployed lines of infantry, and for occasional bayonet charges, which, however, scarcely at any time result in actual hand-to-hand fight, while in villages, farm-yards, intrenchments, &c., the bayonet is often enough actually used. In this open ground, too, the cavalry darts forward whenever opportunities offer themselves, while the artillery continues to play and to advance to new positions. While thus the battle is oscillating, the intentions, the dispositions, and, above all, the strength of the two contending armies are becoming more apparent; more and more troops are engaged, and it soon is shown which party has the strongest body of intact forces in reserve for the final and decisive attack. Either the attacking party has so far been successful, and may now venture to launch his reserve upon the centre or flank of the defending party, or the attack has been so far repulsed and cannot be sustained by fresh troops, in which case the defending party may bring his reserves forward, and by a powerful charge, convert the repulse into a defeat. In most cases, the decisive attack is directed against some part of the enemy's front, in order to break through his line. As much artillery as possible is concentrated upon the chosen point; infantry advances in close masses, and as soon as its charge has proved successful, cavalry dashes into the opening thus made, deploying right and left, taking in flank and rear the enemy's line, and, as the expression is, rolling it up toward its two wings. Such an attack, to be actually decisive, must, however, be undertaken with a large force, and not before the enemy has engaged his last reserves; otherwise the losses incurred would be out of all proportion to the very meagre results to be obtained, and might even cause the loss of the battle. In most cases, a commander will rather break off a battle taking a decidedly unfavorable turn, than engage his last reserves, and wait for the decisive charge of his opponent; and with the present organization and tactics, this may in most cases be done with a comparatively moderate loss, as the enemy after a well-contested battle, is generally in a shattered condition also. The reserves and artillery take a fresh position to the rear, under cover of which the troops are gradually disengaged and retire. It then depends upon the vivacity of the pursuit, whether the retreat be made in good order or not. The enemy will send his cavalry against the troops trying to disengage themselves; and cavalry must, therefore, be at hand to assist them. But if the cavalry of the retiring part be routed and his infantry attained before it is out of reach, then the rout become general, and the rear-guard, in its new defensive position, will have hard work before it unless night is approaching, which is generally the case. Such is the average routine of a modern battle, supposing the parties to be pretty equal in strength and leadership; with a decided superiority on one side, the affair is much abridged, and combinations take place, the variations of which are innumerable; but under all circumstances, modern battles between civilized armies will, on the whole, bear the character above described.

IIE. Engels, 'The Volunteer Movement'*

At the time when the formation of these rifle corps was first agitated, the whole matter savoured very strongly of our own national and civic guards; there was a great deal of playing at soldiers; the way in which officers were manufactured, and the appearance and helplessness of some of these officers, when on duty, were rather amusing. It may well be imagined, the men did not always elect the most capable, or even those who had the movement most at heart. During the first six months, almost all battalions and companies made the same effect upon the beholder as our own defunct civic guard of 1848.

* Excerpts from F. Engels, articles in *Volunteer Journal for Lancashire and Cheshire*, Sept. 14 1860; April 12 1861. [Articles republished in *Engels As Military Critic; Articles by Friedrich Engels reprinted from the Volunteer Journal and the Manchester Guardian of the 1860s*, with an Introduction by W. H. Chaloner and W. O. Henderson (Manchester University Press, 1959).]

This, then, was the material handed over to the drill-sergeants, in order to shape it into a body of serviceable field-troops. The manual and platoon was gone through mostly at nights, between seven and nine o'clock, in covered rooms and by gas-light, twice or three times a week. On Saturday afternoons, if possible, the whole body made a short march and went through company movements. To drill on Sunday was forbidden by both law and custom. The instructors were sergeants and corporals of the line, the militia, or pensioners; and they, too, had to form the officers into shape. But the English non-commissioned officer is an excellent man in his way. There is, on duty, less swearing and coarse language in the English army than in any other; on the other hand, punishment is so much the more certain to be applied. The non-commissioned imitates the commissioned officer, and thus [has] adopted manners far superior to those of our German sergeants. Then he does not serve because of the prospect of some pettifogging office in the civil service being held out to him, as is the case with us; he has engaged himself voluntarily for twelve years, and promotion, up to the rank of sergeant-major even, offers him considerable fresh advantages at every step; in every battalion one or two commissions (adjutant and paymaster) are mostly reserved to old non-commissioned officers; and, on active service, every sergeant may attach the golden star to his collar by distinguishing himself before the enemy. The drill-sergeants belonging to this class of men have, indeed, upon the whole, made the volunteers what it was possible to make them in so short a time; they have not only made them steady in company movements, but also licked the officers into shape.

The men upon the whole looked well. There were, indeed, some companies as puny as Frenchmen, but others surpassed in stature the average of the present British line. Mostly, however, they were very unequal in size and breadth of chest. The pallor peculiar to the inhabitants of towns gave to most of them a rather unpleasantly unwarlike look, but eight days' encampment would soon get the better of that. The uniforms, some of them a little over-ornamental, made a very good effect in the mass.

The first year's drill has taught the volunteers so much of

the elementary movements, that they may now enter upon skirmishing and rifle practice. They will be far more handy at both these kinds of work than the English line, so that by Summer 1861 they would form a very useful army, if only their officers knew more about their business.

This is the weak point of the whole formation. Officers cannot be manufactured in the same time and with the same means as privates. Up to now it has been proved that the willingness and zeal of the mass may be relied upon, as far as is required, for making every man a soldier as far as necessary. But this is not sufficient for the officers. As we have seen, even for simple battalion movements, wheeling in column, deployments, keeping distances (so important in the English system of evolutions, where open columns are very often employed), the officers are not by far sufficiently formed. What is to become of them on outpost and skirmishing duty, where judgement of ground is everything, and where so many other difficult matters are to be taken into consideration? How can such men be entrusted with the duty of taking care of the safety of an army on the march? Government has made it binding upon every officer of volunteers to go to Hythe for three weeks, at least. So far, so good; but that will neither teach him to conduct a patrol, nor to command a picket. And yet, the volunteers are chiefly to be used for light-infantry service—for that very kind of duty which requires the cleverest and most reliable of officers.

But what, it will be said, is the use of such perfection of drill to the volunteers? They are not intended to have it, they cannot be expected to have it, and they will not require it. No doubt this is quite correct. The very attempt to make volunteers emulate the line in perfection of drill would be the ruin of the movement. But drilled the volunteers must be, and so far drilled that common simultaneous action shall become quite mechanical, quite a matter of course with them; so far, that all their movements and motions can be gone through steadily, simultaneously, by all, and with a certain degree of military bearing. In all these points the line will remain the model which they will have to look up to, and company drill will have to be the means by which the required efficiency can alone be obtained.

Take the manual and platoon. That on any given word of command, the whole of the rifles in the battalion should be moved simultaneously, and in the manner prescribed, is not a mere matter of appearance. We must suppose that all volunteer corps are now so far advanced that the men can go through this exercise without positively hurting each other, or knocking their rifles together. But even beyond this, a mere slovenly way of going through the different motions has, undoubtedly, a great moral effect upon the battalion under drill. Why should any one man be particularly attentive to the command, if he has blunders committed right and left, and rifles coming up or down in a straggling way long after he has performed the command? What confidence, before the enemy, can a man on the left wing have in his comrades on the right wing, unless he knows they will load, make ready, and present together with him on the command being given, and will be ready again, as soon as he himself shall be, either to fire again or to charge? Moreover, every experienced soldier will tell you that the habit of such simultaneous action—the certainty of the officer's command being responded to by those two or three round distinct sounds, denoting that every man acts at the same time as his comrades—has a very great moral influence on the battalion. It brings home to the senses of the men the fact that they really are like one body; that they are perfectly in the hand of the commander, and that he can employ their strength at the shortest notice and with the greatest effect.

IIF. Engels, 'The History of the Rifle'*

The wars of the American and French Revolutions created a great change in tactics. Henceforth extended order was introduced in every engagement; the combination of skirmishers with lines or columns became the essential characteristic of modern fighting. The masses, during the greater part of the day, are kept back; they are held in reserve or employed in manœuvring so as to concentrate on the weak point of the enemy; they are only launched in decisive moments; but, in the meantime, skirmishers and their immediate supports

* Excerpts from F. Engels, 'The History of the Rifle', *Volunteer Journal*, Nov. 3 1860; Jan. 5 1861. [Republished in *Engels as Military Critic.*]

are constantly engaged. The mass of the ammunition is spent by them, and the objects they fire at, are seldom larger than the front of a company; in most cases, they have to fire at single men well hidden by covering objects. And yet, the effect of their fire is most important; for every attack is both prepared, and, in the first instance, met by it; they are expected to weaken the resistance of detachments occupying farm houses or villages, as well as to take the edge off the attack of a charging line. Now, with old 'Brown Bess', none of these things could be done effectively. Nobody can ever have been under the fire of skirmishers armed with smooth-bore muskets, without taking home an utter contempt for its efficiency at medium ranges. Still, the rifle in its old shape was not fitted for the mass of skirmishers. The old rifle, in order to facilitate the forcing down of the bullet, must be short, so short that it was but a poor handle to a bayonet; consequently, riflemen were used in such positions only when they were safe against an attack with the bayonet, or by cavalry.

Under these circumstances, the problem at once presented itself; to invent a gun, which combines the range and accuracy of the rifle, with the rapidity and ease of loading, and with the length of barrel of the smooth-bore musket; an arm, which is at the same time a rifle and a handy arm of war, fit to be placed into the hands of every infantry soldier.

Thus we see that with the very introduction of skirmishing into modern tactics, arose the demand for such an improved arm of war. In the nineteenth century, whenever a demand for a thing arises, and that demand be justified by the circumstances of the case, it is sure to be supplied. It was supplied in this case. Almost all improvements in small arms made since 1828 tended to supply it. . . .

When, in modern times, military men and gun-makers were bent upon the construction of a fire-arm which should combine the quick and easy loading of the old musket with the range and precision of the rifle, it was natural that breech-loading should again receive attention. With a proper system of fixing the breech, all difficulties were overcome. The shot, a little larger in diameter than the bore, could then be placed, together with the charge, in the breech, and on being pushed forward by the explosion, would press itself through the bore, fill the grooves with its excess of lead, take the rifling, and exclude all possibility of windage. The only difficulty was the mode of fixing the breech. But what was impossible in the 16th and 17th centuries need not be despaired of now.

The great advantages of a breech-loader, supposing that difficulty overcome, are obvious. The time required for loading is considerably reduced. No drawing, turning round, and returning ramrod. One motion opens the breech, another brings the cartridge into its place, a third closes the breech again. A rapid fire of skirmishers, or a quick succession of volleys, so important in many decisive circumstances, are thus secured in a degree which no muzzle-loader can ever equal. With all muzzle-loaders the art of loading is rendered difficult as soon as the soldier, in skirmishing, is kneeling or laid down behind some covering object. If he keeps behind his shelter he cannot hold his gun in a vertical position, and a great part of his charge will stick on to the sides of the bore while running down; if he holds his gun straight up he has to expose himself. With a breech-loader he can load in any position, even without turning his eye from the enemy, as he can load without looking at his gun. In line, he can load while advancing; pour in volley after volley during the advance, and still arrive upon the enemy with a gun always loaded. The bullet can be of the simplest construction, perfectly solid, and will never run any of the chances by which both compression and expansion shots miss taking the grooves, or experience other unpleasant accidents.

The cleaning of the gun is uncommonly facilitated. The chamber, or place where the powder and bullet lie, which is the part always most exposed to fouling, is here laid completely open and the barrel or tube, open at both ends, can be easily inspected and cleaned to perfection. The parts about the breech being necessarily very heavy, as otherwise they could not withstand the explosion, bring the centre of gravity of the rifle nearer the shoulder, and thereby facilitate a steady aim.

We have seen that the only difficulty consisted in the proper closing of the breech. There can be no doubt that this difficulty has now been fully overcome. The number of breech-loaders brought out during the last twenty years is wonderful, and some of them, at least, fulfil all reasonable expections, both as to the efficiency and solidity of the breech-loading apparatus, and as to the ease and rapidity with which the breech can be fixed and unfixed. . . .

The needle-gun was invented by a civilian, Mr. Dreyse, of Sömmerda, in Prussia. After having first invented the method of firing a gun by means of a needle suddenly penetrating an explosive substance fixed in the cartridge, he completed his invention, as early as 1835, by constructing a breech-loader, supplied with this needle-firing apparatus. The Prussian Government at once bought up the secret, and succeeded in keeping it to themselves up to 1848, when it became public; in the meantime they resolved upon giving this arm, in case of war, to all their infantry, and commenced manufacturing needle-guns. At present, the whole infantry of the line, and the greater portion of the Landwehr are armed with it, while all the light cavalry are at this moment receiving breech-loading needle-carbines. . . .

The introduction into an army of an arm capable of such rapid firing will necessarily produce many speculations as to what changes this will produce in tactics; especially among people so fond of speculating as the North Germans. There has been no end of controversies on the pretended revolution in tactics which the needle-gun was to produce. The majority of the military public, in Prussia, at last came to the result that no charge could be made against a battalion firing needle-gun volleys in rapid succession, and that consequently it was all up with the bayonet. If this foolish notion had prevailed, the needle-gun would have brought upon the Prussians many a severe defeat. Fortunately, the Italian war proved to all who could see, that the fire from modern rifles is not necessarily so very dangerous to a battalion charging with spirit, and Prince Frederick Charles of Prussia has taken occasion therefrom to remind his comrades that passive defence, if ever so well armed, is always sure of defeat. The tide of military opinion has turned. People again begin to see that men, and not muskets, must win battles; and if any real change in tactics will be made by the new gun, it will be a return to a greater use of deployed lines (where the ground admits of it), and even to that charge in line which, after having won most of the battles of Frederick the Great, had become almost unknown to the Prussian infantry.

IIG. Marx and Engels, 'The American Civil War'*

March 26 1862.—From whatever standpoint one regards it, the American Civil War presents a spectacle without parallel in the annals of military history. The vast extent of the disputed territory; the far-flung fronts of the lines of operation; the numerical strength of the hostile armies, whose creation derived barely any support from previous organizational bases; the fabulous costs of these armies; the manner of their administration and the general tactical and strategic principles with which the war is waged—all these are new in the eyes of the European onlooker.

The Secessionist conspiracy, organized long before its outbreak, protected and supported by Buchanan's administration, gave the South an advantage by which alone it could hope to achieve its aim. Endangered by its slave population and by a strong Unionist element among the whites themselves, with a population of free men one-third the size of the North, but more ready to attack, thanks to the multitude of adventurous idlers that it harbors—for the South, everything depended on a swift, bold, almost foolhardy offensive. If the Southerners succeeded in capturing St. Louis, Cincinnati, Washington, Baltimore, and perhaps also Philadelphia, they could count on a panic, during which diplomacy and bribery could secure recognition of the independence of all the slave states. If this first attack failed, at least at the decisive points, their position must worsen daily, simultaneously with the development of the strength of the North. This point was correctly understood by the men who had organized the secessionist conspiracy in a truly Bonapartist spirit. They opened the campaign in a corresponding manner. Their bands of adventurers overran Missouri and Tennessee, while their more regular troops invaded East Virginia and prepared a *coup de main* against Washington. With the miscarriage of this coup, the Southern campaign was lost *from a military standpoint.*

The North came to the theater of war reluctantly, sleepily,

* Excerpts from K. Marx and F. Engels, articles in *Die Presse* (Vienna), March 26, 27, and May 30, 1862. [Translated in K. Marx, *On America and the Civil War*, ed. and trans. by S. K. Padover (New York: McGraw Hill, 1972).]

as was to be expected from its higher industrial and commercial development. The social machinery was incomparably more complicated here than in the South, and it required far more time to give its movement this unaccustomed direction. The enlistment of three-month volunteers was a great, but perhaps unavoidable, mistake. It was the policy of the North first to remain on the defensive at all decisive points, to organize its forces, to train them through operations on a small scale and without risking decisive battles, and finally, as soon as the organization was sufficiently strengthened and the traitorous element was at the same time more or less removed from the army, to pass to an energetic, unrelenting offensive and, above all, to reconquer Kentucky, Tennessee, Virginia, and North Carolina. The transformation of citizens into soldiers was bound to take more time in the North than in the South. Once effected, one could count on the individual superiority of the Northern man.

By and large, and allowing for the mistakes that sprang more from political than from military sources, the North acted in accordance with those principles. The guerrilla warfare in Missouri and West Virginia, while it protected the Unionist populations, accustomed the troops to field service and to fire, without exposing them to decisive defeats. The great disgrace of Bull Run was to some extent the result of the earlier mistake of enlisting volunteers for three months. It was senseless to allow a strong position, on difficult terrain, possessed by an enemy hardly inferior in numbers, to be attacked by raw recruits in the front lines. The panic which took possession of the Union Army at the decisive moment—and its cause has not yet been clarified—could surprise no one who was to some extent familiar with the history of people's wars. Such things happened very often to the French troops in 1792-95, but nevertheless did not prevent them from winning the battles of Jemappes and Fleurus, Montenotte, Castiglione, and Rivoli. The jokes of the European press over the Bull Run panic had only one excuse for their silliness—the previous bragging of a part of the North American press.

The six months' respite that followed the defeat at Manassas was utilized by the North better than by the South. Not only were the Northern ranks filled up in greater measure than the

Southern ones. Their officers received better instructions; the discipline and training of the troops did not encounter the same obstacles as in the South. Traitors and incompetents were more and more removed, and the period of the Bull Run panic already belongs to the past. The armies on both sides are, of course, not to be measured by the standard of great European armies or even by that of the former Regular Army of the United States. Napoleon could in fact drill battalions of raw recruits in the depots during the first month, have them march during the second month, and lead them against the enemy during the third month; but then every battalion received a sufficient stiffening of officers and noncommissioned officers, every company some old soldiers, and on the day of battle the new troops were brigaded together with veterans and, so to speak, framed by them. All these conditions were lacking in America. Without the considerable mass of military experience that emigrated to America as a result of the European revolutionary commotions of 1848-49, the organization of the Union Army would have required even a much longer time. The very small number of killed and wounded in proportion to the sum total of the troops engaged (usually one out of twenty) proves that most of the engagements, even the most recent ones in Kentucky and Tennessee, were mainly fought with firearms at fairly long range, and that the occasional bayonet attacks either soon stopped before the enemy fire or put the enemy to flight before it came to hand-to-hand encounter.

March 27 1862.—The leadership of the Kentucky campaign from Somerset to Nashville deserves the highest praise. The reconquest of so extensive a territory, the advance from the Ohio to the Cumberland in a single month, shows an energy, decisiveness, and speed that have seldom been attained by the regular armies of Europe. One compares, for example, the slow advance of the Allies from Magenta to Solferino in the year 1859—without pursuit of the retreating enemy, without endeavour to cut off his stragglers or in any way to envelop and encircle whole bodies of his troops.

Halleck and Grant in particular offer fine examples of decisive military leadership. Without the slightest regard for either Columbus or Bowling Green, they concentrated their forces at the decisive points, Fort Henry and Fort Donelson, captured them quickly and energetically, and thereby made Columbus and Bowling Green untenable. Then they promptly marched on Clarksville and Nashville, without giving the retreating Secessionists time to take up new positions in North Tennessee. During this rapid pursuit the corps of Secessionist troops in Columbus was completely cut off from the center and right wing of its army. English papers have criticized this operation unjustly. Even if the attack on Fort Donelson had failed, the Secessionists, kept busy by General Buell in Bowling Green, could not have detached sufficient men to enable the garrison to follow the repulsed Unionists into open country or to endanger their retreat. Columbus, on the other hand, was so far away that it could not interfere at all with Grant's movements. In fact, after the Unionists had cleared Missouri of the Secessionists, Columbus became an entirely useless post for the latter. The troops who constituted their garrison had to greatly hasten their retreat to Memphis or even to Arkansas. to escape the danger of an inglorious laying down of their arms.

In consequence of the clearing of Missouri and the reconquest of Kentucky, the theater of war has so far narrowed that the various armies can to a certain extent cooperate along the whole line of operations to achieve definite results. In other words, the war only now assumes a *strategic* character, and the geographic configuration of the country acquires a new interest. It is now the task of the Northern generals to find the Achilles heel of the cotton states. . . .

The American newspapers influenced by McClellan are making a great to-do over the anaconda-like envelopment theory. According to this, a vast line of armies is to envelop the rebels, gradually constrict its coils, and finally strangle the enemy. This is pure childishness. It is a rehash of the so-called *Cordon* system, invented in Austria around 1770, which was employed against the French from 1792 to 1797 with such great stubbornness and such constant failure. At Jemappes, Fleurus, and particularly at Montenotte, Millesimo, Dego, Castiglione, and Rivoli, the knockout blow was dealt to this system. The French cut the 'anaconda' in two by attacking at a point where they had concentrated superior forces. Then the pieces of the 'anaconda' were chopped to bits one after another.

In well-populated and more or less centralized states, there is always a center whose occupation by the enemy would break the national resistance. Paris is a shining example. But the slave states possess no such center. They are sparsely populated, with few big cities and all of these on the seacoast. One therefore asks: Does there, nevertheless, exist a military center of gravity whose capture would break the backbone of their resistance, or are they, as Russia still was in 1812, unconquerable without, in a word, occupying every village and every patch of ground along the whole periphery?

Cast a glance at the geographic configuration of Secessia, with its long coastline on the Atlantic Ocean and its long coastline on the Gulf of Mexico. So long as the Confederates held Kentucky and Tennessee, the whole formed a great compact mass. The loss of those two states drives an immense wedge into their territory, separating the states on the North Atlantic Ocean from those on the Gulf of Mexico. The direct route from Virginia and the two Carolinas to Texas, Louisiana, Mississippi, and partly even to Alabama leads through Tennessee, which is now occupied by the Unionists. The *only* route, after the complete capture of Tennessee by the Union, that links the two sections of the slave states goes through Georgia. This proves that *Georgia is the key to Secessia.* With the loss of Georgia, the Confederacy would be cut into two sections which would have lost all connection with each other. . . .

Would the conquest of all of Georgia, together with the seacoast of Florida, be required for such an operation? By no means. In a land where communication, particularly between distant points, depends much more on railroads than on highways, the seizure of railroads suffices.

May 30 1862.—McClellan has proved indisputably that he is a military incompetent who, having been elevated by favorable circumstances to a commanding and responsible position, wages war not in order to defeat the enemy, but rather in order not to be defeated by the enemy and thereby forfeit his own usurped greatness. He comports himself like the old so-called 'maneuvering generals,' who excused their anxious avoidance of any tactical decision on the ground that by strategic envelopment they forced the enemy to give up his positions. The Confederates always escape him, because at the decisive moment he never attacks them. Thus—although their plan of retreat had already been announced ten days before, even in the New York papers (for example, the *Tribune*)—he let them quietly retire from Manassas to Richmond. Then he divided his army and flanked the Confederates strategically, while with one body of troops he established himself before Yorktown. A war of sieges always affords a pretext for wasting time and avoiding battle. No sooner had he concentrated a military force superior to that of the Confederates than he let them retire from Yorktown to Williamsburg and from there farther, without forcing them to join battle. Never has a war been waged so wretchedly. If the rear-guard action near Williamsburg ended in defeat for the troops of the Confederate rear instead of a second Bull Run for the Union troops, McClellan was entirely innocent of this result. . . .

The Confederate army in Virginia has better chances than Beauregard's army, first because it is facing a McClellan instead of a Halleck, and second, because the many rivers on its line of retreat flow crosswise from the mountains to the sea. Nevertheless, in order to avoid being broken up into bands *without a battle*, its generals will be forced sooner or later to accept a decisive battle, exactly as the Russians had to fight at Smolensk and Borodino against the best judgement of the generals. Wretched as McClellan's generalship has been, the constant retreats, accompanied by abandonment of artillery, munitions, and other military supplies, and simultaneously the small, unlucky rearguard actions—all these have in any case badly demoralized the Confederates, as will become evident on the day of a decisive battle. We come, therefore, to the summary:

If Beauregard or Jefferson Davis should lose a decisive battle, his armies would dissolve into bands. If one of them should win a decisive battle, which is altogether improbable, the dissolution of their armies would at best be deferred. They are in no position to make even the slightest lasting use of a victory. They cannot advance twenty English miles without coming to a standstill and again awaiting a renewed enemy offensive.

It still remains to examine the chances of a guerrilla war. But it is precisely in this war of the slaveholders that it is most amazing how little, or rather how nonexistent, has been the participation of the population. In the year 1813 the communications of the French were constantly interrupted and harrassed by Colomb, Lützow, Chernyshev, and twenty other leaders of insurgents and Cossacks. In 1812 the Russian population completely vanished before the French line of march; in 1814 the French peasants armed themselves and killed the patrols and stragglers of the Allies; but here nothing happens at all. People resign themselves to the fortune of the big battles and console themselves with '*Victrix causa diis placuit, sed victa Catoni.*'* The boast about the war at sea dissolves into vapor. There can hardly be any doubt, to be sure, that the 'white trash,' as the planters themselves call the poor whites, will attempt guerrilla warfare and brigandage. But such an attempt will very quickly transform the property-owning planters into Unionists. They themselves will call the troops of the Yankees to their aid. The alleged burnings of cotton, etc., on the Mississippi rest exclusively on the testimony of two Kentuckians, who are said to have come to Louisville—surely not up the Mississippi. The conflagration in New Orleans was easily organized. The fanaticism of the New Orleans merchants is explained on the ground that they were obliged to take a mass of Confederate Treasury bonds for hard cash. The conflagration at New Orleans will be repeated in other cities; assuredly there will be some other burnings. but such theatrical coups can only bring the split between the planters and the 'white trash' to a head, and therewith, *finis Secessiae!*

IIH. Engels, 'The Seven Weeks' War'**

June 20 1866.—The Prussian soldiers, especially the men of the reserve and such Landwehr men as had to be taken to fill up vacancies in the line (and there are many) go to war, against their will; the Austrians, on the contrary, have long wished for a war with Prussia, and await with impatience the order

* 'The victorious cause was pleasing to the gods, but that of the vanquished to Cato.'

** Excerpts from F. Engels's articles in *Manchester Guardian*, June 20, July 3, 6, 1866. [Articles republished in *Engels as Military Critic*.]

to move. They have, therefore, also the advantage in the *morale* of the troops.

Prussia has had no great war for fifty years; her army is, on the whole, a peace army, with the pedantry and martinetism inherent to all peace armies. No doubt a great deal has been done latterly, especially since 1859, to get rid of this; but the habits of forty years are not so easily eradicated, and a great number of incapable and pedantic men must still be found, particularly in the most important places—those of the field officers. Now the Austrians have been fundamentally cured of this complaint by the war of 1859, and have turned their dearly-bought experience to the very best use. No doubt, in organization of detail, in adaptation, for, and experience in, warfare, the Austrians again are superior to the Prussians.

With the exception of the Russians the Prussians are the only troops whose normal formation for fighting is the deep close column. Imagine the eight companies of an English battalion in a quarter-distance column, but two companies instead of one forming the front, so that four rows of two companies each form the column, and you have the 'Prussian column of attack'. A better target for rifled fire-firms than this could not be imagined, and, since rifled cannon can throw a shell into it at 2,000 yards range, such a formation must render it almost impossible to reach the enemy at all. Let one single shell explode in the midst of this mass, and see whether that battalion is fit for anything afterwards on that day.

The Austrians have adopted the loose open column of the French, which is scarcely to be called a column; it is more like two or three lines following each other at 20 or 30 yards distance, and is scarcely, if anything more exposed to losses by artillery than a deployed line. The advantage of tactical formation is, again, on the side of the Austrians.

Against all these advantages the Prussians have but two points to set off. Their commissariat is decidedly better, and the troops will therefore be better fed. The Austrian commissariat, like all Austrian administration, is one den of bribery and peculation scarcely better than in Russia. Even now we hear of the troops being badly and irregularly fed in the field and in the fortresses it will be worse still, and the Austrian Administration may happen to be a more dangerous enemy to the fortresses in the Quadrilateral than the Italian artillery.

The second set-off the Prussians have is their superior armament. Although their rifled artillery is decidedly better than that of the Austrians, this will make very little difference in the open field. The range, trajectory, and accuracy of the Prussian and Austrian rifles will be about on a par; but the Prussians have breech-loaders, and can deliver a steady well-aimed fire in the ranks at least four times a minute. The immense superiority of this arm has been proved in the Danish war, and there is no doubt the Austrians will experience it in a far higher degree. If they, as it is said Benedek has instructed them to do, will not lose much time with firing, but go at the enemy at once with the bayonet, they will have enormous losses. In the Danish war, the loss of the Prussians was never more than one fourth, sometimes only one tenth, of that of the Danes; and, as a military correspondent of *The Times* a short time ago very correctly pointed out, the Danes were almost everywhere beaten by a minority of troops actually engaged.

Still, in spite of the needle gun, the odds are against the Prussians; and if they refuse to be beaten in the first great battle by the superior leadership, organization, tactical formation, and *morale* of the Austrians, and last, not least, by their own commanders, then they must certainly be of a different mettle from that of which a peace army of 50 years' standing may be expected to be.

July 3 1866.–Suppose a young Prussian ensign or cornet, under examination for a lieutenancy, to be asked what would be the safest plan for a Prussian army to invade Bohemia? Suppose our young officer were to answer,–'Your best way will be to divide your troops into two about equal bodies, to send one round by the east of the Riesengebirge, the other to the west, and effect their junction in Gitschin.' What would the examining officer say to this? He would inform the young gentleman that this plan sinned against the two very first laws of strategy: Firstly, never to divide your troops so that they cannot support each other, but to keep them well together; and, secondly, in case of an advance on different roads, to effect the junction of the different columns at a point which is not within reach of the enemy; that, therefore, the plan proposed was the very worst of all; that it could only be taken into consideration at all in case Bohemia was quite unoccupied by hostile troops, and that, consequently, an officer proposing such a plan of campaign was not fit to hold even a lieutenant's commission.

Yet, this is the very plan which the wise and learned staff of the Prussian army have adopted. It is almost incredible; but it is so. The mistake for which the Italians had to suffer at Custozza, has been again committed by the Prussians, and under circumstances which made it ten-fold worse. The Italians knew at least that, with ten divisions, they would be numerically superior to the enemy. The Prussians must have known that if they kept their nine corps together they would be at best barely on a par, as far as numbers went, with Benedek's eight corps; and that by dividing their troops they exposed the two armies to the almost certain fate of being crushed in succession by superior numbers. It would be completely inexplicable how such a plan could ever by discussed, much less adopted, by a body of such unquestionably capable officers as form the Prussian staff—if it was not for the fact of King William being in chief command. But nobody could possibly expect that the fatal consequences of kings and princes taking high command would come out so soon and so strong. . . .

The Prussians must have behaved splendidly for an old peace army. When war was actually declared, a totally different spirit came over the army, brought on, chiefly, by the clearing-out of the small fry of potentates in the north-west. It gave the troops—rightly or wrongly, we merely register the fact—the idea that they were asked to fight, this time, for the unification of Germany, and the hitherto sullen and sulky men of the reserve and Landwehr then crossed the frontier of Austria with loud cheers. It is owing to this chiefly that they fought so well; but at the same time we must ascribe the greater portion of whatever success they have had to their breech-loaders; and if they ever get out of the difficulties into which their generals so wantonly placed them, they will have to thank the needle-gun for it. The reports as to its immense superiority over the muzzle-loaders are again unanimous. A sergeant from the Martini regiment, taken prisoner, said to the correspondent of the *Cologne Gazette*: 'We have surely done whatever may be expected from brave soldiers, but no man can stand against that rapid fire.' If the Austrians are beaten, it will be not so much General Benedek or General Ramming as General Ramrod who is to blame for the result....

July 6 1866.–No doubt the needle-gun, with its rapid fire, has done a great part of this. It may be doubted whether without it the junction of the two Prussian armies could have been effected; and it is quite certain that this immense and rapid success could not have been obtained without such superior fire, for the Austrian army is habitually less subject to panic than most European armies. But there were other circumstances co-operating. We have already mentioned the excellent dispositions and unhesitating action of the two Prussian armies, from the moment they entered Bohemia. We may add that they also deviated, in this campaign, from the column system, and brought their masses forward principally in deployed lines, so as to bring every rifle into activity, and to save their men from the fire of artillery. We must acknowledge that the movements both on the march and before the enemy were carried out with an order and punctuality which no man could have expected from an army and administration covered with the rust of fifty years' peace. And, finally, all the world must have been surprised at the dash displayed by these young troops in each and every engagement without exception. It is all very well to say the breech-loaders did it, but they are not self-acting, they want stout hearts and strong arms to carry them. The Prussians fought very often against superior numbers, and were almost everywhere the attacking party; the Austrians, therefore, had the choice of ground. And in attacking strong positions and barricaded towns, the advantages of the breech loader almost disappear; the bayonet has to do the work, and there has been a good deal of it. The cavalry, moreover, acted with the same dash, and with them cold steel and speed of horses are the only weapons in a charge. The French *canards* of Prussian cavalry lines first peppering their opponents with carbine fire (breech-loading or otherwise) and then rushing at them sword in hand, could only originate among a people whose cavalry has very often been guilty of that trick, and always been punished for it by being borne down by the superior impetus of the charging enemy. There is no mistaking it, the Prussian army has, within a single week, conquered a position as high as ever it held, and may well feel confident now to be able to cope with any opponent. There is no campaign on record where an equally signal success, in an equally short time, and without any noteworthy check, has been obtained, except that campaign of Jena which annihilated the Prussians of that day, and, if we except the defeat of Ligny, the campaign of Waterloo.

IIJ. Trotsky, 'Engels as Military Thinker'*

Friedrich Engels' book is, for the most part, an analytical chronicle of the Franco-Prussian War of 1870–71. It is composed of articles published in the English *Pall Mall Gazette* during the war events. This is enough to make it clear that the reader cannot count on finding in these articles a sort of monograph on war or any systematic presentation of the theory of the art of war. No, Engels' task consisted—proceeding from the general appraisal of the forces and means of the two adversaries and following from day to day the manner of employing these forces and means—in helping the reader orient himself in the course of the military operations and even in lifting the so-called veil of the future a little from time to time. . . .

It is clear that a book of this kind cannot be read and studied like the other, purely theoretical, works of Engels. To understand perfectly the ideas and evaluations of a concrete, factual kind contained in this book, all the operations of the Franco-Prussian War must be followed step by step on the map, and the viewpoints set forth in the latest war-historical literature taken into consideration. The average reader cannot of course set himself the task of such a critical-scientific labor: it calls for military training, a great expenditure of time and special interest in the subject. But would such interest be justified? In our opinion, Yes. It is justified primarily from the standpoint of a correct evaluation of the military level and the

*Excerpts from Trotsky's review of Engels, *Notes on War* in 'Marxism and Military Warfare', *Military Writings*, March 19 1924, pp. 134 f., 140–5.

military perspicacity of Friedrich Engels himself. A thorough examination of Engels' extremely concise text, the comparison of his judgments and prognoses made at the same time by military writers of the time, could count on attracting great interest, and would not only be a valuable contribution to the biography of Engels—and his biography is an important chapter in the history of socialism—but also as an extremely apt illustration in the question of the reciprocal relations between Marxism and the military profession.

Of Marxism or dialectics, Engels says not a word in all these articles; which is not to be astonished at, for he was writing anonymously for an arch-bourgeois periodical and that at a time when the name of Marx was still little known. But only these outward reasons prompted Engels to refrain from all general-theoretical considerations. We may be convinced that even if Engels had had the opportunity then to discuss the events of the war in a revolutionary-Marxian paper—with far greater freedom for expressing his political sympathies and antipathies—he would nevertheless hardly have approached the analysis and the estimation of the course of the war differently than he did in the *Pall Mall Gazette.* Engels injected no abstract doctine into the domain of the science of war from without and did not set up any tactical recipes, newly-discovered by himself, as universal criteria.

Regardless of the conciseness of the presentation, we see nonetheless with what attentiveness the author deals with all the elements of the profession of war, from the territorial areas and the population figures of the countries involved down to the biographical researches into the past of General Trochu for the purpose of being better acquainted with his methods and habits. Behind these articles is sensed a vast preceding and continuing labor. . . .

In some passages, Engels mentions fleetingly the harmful effect that the penetration of 'politics' can have in the course of war operations. This observation of his seems at first blush to be in conflict with the conception that war, by and large, is nothing but a continuation of politics. In reality, there is no contradiction here. The war continues politics, but with special means and methods. When politics is compelled, for the solution of its fundamental tasks, to resort to the aid of war, this politics must not hamper the course of the war operations for the sake of its subordinated tasks. When Bonaparte took actions which were obviously inexpedient from the military standpoint in order, as Engels opines, to influence 'public opinion' favorably with ephemeral successes, this was undoubtedly to be regarded as an inadmissable invasion of politics into the conduct of the war which made it impossible for the latter to accomplish the fundamental tasks set by politics. To the degree that Bonaparte was forced, in the struggle to preserve his régime, to permit such an invasion of politics, an obvious self-condemnation of the régime was revealed which made the early collapse inevitable. . . .

Engels has an excellent knowledge of where, given all the other necessary pre-conditions, the main difficulties lie in transforming a human mass into a company or a battalion. 'Whoever,' says he, 'has seen popular levies on the drill-ground or under fire—be they Baden Freischaaren, Bull-Run Yankees, French Mobiles, or British Volunteers—will have perceived at once that the chief cause of the helplessness and unsteadiness of these troops lies in the fact of the officers not knowing their duty.'

It is most instructive to see how attentively Engels treats the home guards of an army. How far removed this great revolutionist is from all the pseudo-revolutionary chatter which was very popular in France right at that time—on the saving power of a mass mobilization (*levée en masse*), an armed nation (armed in a trice), etc. Engels knows very well the great importance officers and non-commissioned officers have in a battalion. He makes exact calculations on what resources in officers have remained to the republic following the defeat of the regular forces of the Empire. He gives the greatest attention to the development of those features in the new, so-called Loire army which distinguish it from armed human mass. Thus, for example, he records with satisfaction that the new army not only intends to proceed unitedly and to obey orders, but also that it 'has learned again one very important thing which Louis Napoleon's army had quite forgotten—light infantry duty, the art of protecting flanks and rear from surprise, of feeling for the enemy, surprising his detachments, procuring information and prisoners.'

This is how Engels is everywhere in his 'newspaper' articles: bold in his grasp of affairs, realistic in method, perspicacious in big things and little, and always scrupulous in the manipulation of materials. He counts the number of drawn and smooth-bore gun barrels of the French, repeatedly checks on the German artillery, thinks of the qualities of the Prussian cavalry horse, and never forgets the qualities of the Prussian non-commissioned officer. Faced in the course of events by the problem of the siege and defense of Paris, he investigates the quality of its fortifications, the strength of the artillery of the Germans and the French, and takes up very critically the question of whether there are regular troops behind the walls of Paris that may be called effective for battle. What a pity we did not have this work of Engels in 1918! It would surely have helped us overcome more speedily and easily the then widely disseminated prejudice with which it was sought to counterpose 'revolutionary enthusiasm' and the 'proletarian spirit' to a professional organization, flawless discipline and trained command. . . .

Relentlessly ruling out of his analysis every abstraction, regarding war as a material chain of operations, considering every operation from the standpoint of the actually existing forces, means and the possibility of employing them, this great revolutionist acts as . . . a war specialist, that is, as a person who by mere virtue of his profession or his vocation proceeds from the internal factors of the conduct of war. It is not astonishing that Engels' articles were attributed to renowned military men of the time, which led to Engels' being nicknamed the 'General' among his circle of friends. Yes, he handled military questions like a 'general,' perhaps not without substantial defects in specific military domains and without the necessary practical experience, but, in exchange, with a talented head such as not every general has on his shoulders.

But, it might be asked, where, after all this, is Marxism? To this may be replied that it is precisely here—up to a certain degree—that it is expressed. One of the fundamental philosophical premises of Marxism says that the truth is always concrete. This means that the profession of war and its problems cannot be dissolved into social and political categories. War is war, and the Marxist who wants to judge it must bear in mind that the truth of war is also concrete. And this is what Engels' book teaches primarily. But not this alone.

If military problems may not be dissolved into general political problems, it is likewise impermissible to separate the latter from the former. As we have already mentioned, war is a continuation of politics by special means. This profoundly dialectical thought was formulated by Clausewitz. War is a continuation of politics: whoever wishes to understand the 'continuation' must get clear on what preceded it. But continuation—'by other means'—signifies: it is not enough to be well oriented politically in order to be able therewith also to estimate correctly the 'other means' of war. The greatest and incomparable merit of Engels consisted in the fact that while he had a profound grasp of the independent character of war—with its own inner technique, structure, its methods, traditions and prejudices—he was at the same time a great expert in politics, to which war is in the last analysis subordinated.

It need not be said that this tremendous superiority could not guarantee Engels against mistakes in his concrete military judgements and prognoses. During the Civil War in the United States, Engels overrated the purely military superiority that the Southerners displayed in the first period and was therefore inclined to believe in their victory. During the German-Austrian War in 1866, shortly before the decisive battle at Königgrätz, which laid the foundation stone for the predominance of Prussia, Engels counted on a mutiny in the Prussian Landwehr. In the chronicle of the Franco-Prussian War, too, a number of mistakes in isolated matters can undoubtedly be found, even though the general prognosis of Engels in this case was incomparably more correct than in the two examples adduced. Only very naïve persons can think that the greatness of a Marx, Engels or Lenin consists in the automatic infallibility of all their judgments. No, they too made mistakes. But in judging the greatest and most complicated questions they used to make fewer mistakes than all the others. And therein is shown the greatness of their thinking. And also in the fact that their mistakes, when the reasons for them are seriously examined, often proved to be deeper and more instructive than the correct judgement of those who, accidentally or not, were right as against them in this or that case.

Abstractions of all kinds, such as that every class *must* have specific tactics and strategy peculiar to itself, naturally find no support in Engels. He knows all too well that the foundation of all foundations of a military organization and a war is determined by the level of the development of the productive forces and not by the naked class will. To be sure, it may be said that the feudal epoch had its own tactics and even a number of coördinated tactics, that the bourgeois epoch, in turn, has known not one but several tactics, and that socialism will surely lead to the elaboration of new war tactics if it is forced into the position of having to coexist with capitalism for a long time. Stated in this general form it is correct, in the degree that the level of the productive forces of capitalist society is higher than that of feudal, and in the socialist society it will with time be still higher. But nothing further than this. For it in no wise follows that the proletariat which has attained power and disposes of only a very low level of production, can immediately form new tactics which—in principle—can only flow from the enhanced development of the productive forces of the future socialist society.

In the past we have very often compared economic processes and phenomena with military. Now it will perhaps not be without value to counterpose some military questions to the economic, for in the latter domain we have already garnered a fairly considerable experience. The most important part of industry is working with us under conditions of socialist economy, by virtue of the fact that it is the property of the workers' state and produces on its account and under its direction. By virtue of this circumstance, the social-juridical structure of our industry is incisively distinguished from the capitalistic. This finds its expression in the system of administration of industry, in the election of the directing personnel, in the relationship between the factory management and the workers, etc. But how do matters stand with the process of production itself? Have we perhaps created our own socialist methods of production, which are counterposed to the capitalistic? We are still a long distance from that. The methods of production depend upon the material technique and the cultural and productive level of the workers. Given the worn-out installations and inadequate utilization of our plant, the production process now stands on an incomparably lower level than before the war. In this field we have not only created nothing new, but we can only hope after a number of years to acquire those methods and means of production which are at present introduced into the advanced capitalist countries and which assure them thereby of a far higher productivity of labor. If, however, this is how matters stand in the field of economy, how can it be otherwise in principle in the military field? Tactics depend upon the existing war technique and the military and cultural level of the soldiers.

To be sure, the political and social-juridical structure of our army is basically different from the bourgeois armies. This is expressed in the selection of the commanding personnel, in the relationship between it and the soldier-mass, and primarily in the political aims that inspire our army. But in no wise does it follow from this that now, on the basis of our low technical and cultural level, we are already able to create tactics, new in principle and more perfected, than those which the most civilized beasts of prey of the West have attained. The first steps of the proletariat which has conquered power—and these first steps are measured in years—must not—as the same Engels taught—be confused with the socialist society, which stands on a higher stage of development. In accordance with the growth of the productive forces on the basis of socialist property, our production process itself will also necessarily assume a different character than under capitalism. In order to change the character of production qualitatively, we need no more revolutions, no shakeups in property, etc.: we need only a development of the productive forces on the foundation already created. The same applies also to the army. In the Soviet state, on the basis of a working community between workers and peasants, under the direction of the advanced workers, we shall undoubtedly create new tactics. But when? When our productive forces outstrip the capitalistic, or at least approximate them.

III. CAPITALISM, SOCIALISM, AND MILITARISM

In the view of such twentieth-century Marxist theorists as Luxemburg, Bukharin, Lenin, and Mandel, economic necessities had compelled capitalism to turn to war and to imperial expansion in order to relieve the internal problems to which the system gave rise. Rosa Luxemburg (1870–1919), a Polish-born economist, was one of the leaders of the Left-wing German socialists, most particularly during and immediately after the war of 1914. (She was peremptorily executed by armed units in the suppression of communist agitation against the post-war Socialist government.) In the essay (Section IIIA, 1) on 'Militarism as a Province of Accumulation', written in 1913, Luxemburg argued that only by the manufacture of armaments could capitalism employ that surplus portion of the income created by the system which would otherwise so disturb the circulation of wealth as to produce industrial crises and widespread unemployment.

The Russian Marxist economist, Nikolai Bukharin (1880–1938) in 1915, depicted capitalism as 'unthinkable without armaments . . . [and] without wars'. (Section IIIA, 2.) Bukharin described a neo-mercantile capitalism characterized by the predominance of trusts which required considerable military establishments to defend their interests. In this analysis, he owed much to Luxemburg, and much as well to the ideas of the German economist Rudolf Hilferding (1871–1941). Bukharin (who served as Arthur Koestler's model for the character Rubashov in *Darkness at Noon*) was tried and executed in the purge of the late thirties.

Most notably, the leader of the Bolshevik Revolution, V. I. Lenin, in a highly influential tract written in 1917 on *Imperialism*, followed the analysis of the English liberal J. A. Hobson as well as Hilferding. He portrayed a capitalism which had come to its last stage of development. In an effort to secure higher rates of profit, the capitalists were dividing up the non-European world to exploit its labour and natural resources. The relative strength of the great powers was always undergoing change, and nations would always seek a reapportionment of the spoils of empire. Consequently, war, Lenin insisted, was the leading characteristic of this late capitalism (Section IIIA, 3). (This remains the view of the makers of contemporary Soviet doctrine; see sections V, A–G.) Lastly, a present-day Belgian Marxist economist, Ernest Mandel, argues much like his predecessors, though bringing them somewhat up to date by examining in some detail such phenomena as the modern war economy, what he calls 'the permanent tendency to currency inflation'. (Section IIIA, 4.).

In this section, we also include a number of further writings on Marxism and war written by Lenin. V. I. Lenin (1870–1924) was the founder of the Bolshevik faction of the Russian Social Democratic Party and the leader of the successful Revolution which overthrew the Kerensky regime in October 1917. Lenin's elder brother, Alexander, had been executed in 1881 for his part in the assassination of the Tsar, and Lenin followed him into the revolutionary movement. After two terms in Siberian prison camps, Lenin left Russia for Switzerland in 1900, returning briefly to take part in the unsuccessful revolt of 1905. After the outbreak of the revolution of March 1917, German military authorities returned Lenin to Russia in a sealed box-car in the expectation that he would help to disrupt the Russian war effort. Soon after coming to power, he and Trotsky made peace with Germany. After his death, Lenin was virtually apotheosized by the Bolsheviks, and his version of communist doctrine, Marxism–Leninism, became the ideological base of the Soviet state.

In 1915 and 1916, before the Revolution, Lenin attempted to distinguish between a Marxist view of the war, one which saw in the international conflict an opportunity for world revolution, and that of a liberal and pacifist bourgeoisie. (Sections IIIC, 1; B, 1c.) He urged the creation of a proletarian militia, which was actually formed after the bourgeois March revolution, and which assisted in making the Bolshevik Revolution of October 1917. (Section IIIB, 1b.) In another work of these pre-revolutionary years, Lenin insisted that a dictatorship of the proletariat could only be maintained by armed troops. (Section IIIC, 1.) Leon Trotsky (in Section IIIC, 2a, b) agreed, stressing the importance of Bolsheviks learning the traditional military doctrine, rather than striving after the fantasy of creating a proletarian science of war. Mao (Section IIIC, 3) much like Lenin declared that 'Political power grows out of the barrel of a gun', a view he described as properly Marxist. In the final selection, we observe that recent Soviet military theorists continue to hold to this general line. (Section IIIC 4; for a note on Byely, see Introductory Remarks to Section I.)

IIIA. The Inevitability of War Under Capitalism

*1. Rosa Luxemburg, 'Militarism as a Province of Accumulation'**

Militarism fulfils a quite definite function in the history of capital, accompanying as it does every historical phase of accumulation. It plays a decisive part in the first stages of European capitalism, in the period of the so-called 'primitive accumulation', as a means of conquering the New World and the spice-producing countries of India. Later, it is employed to subject the modern colonies, to destroy the social organisations of primitive societies so that their means of production may be appropriated, forcibly to introduce commodity trade in countries where the social structure had been unfavourable to it, and to turn the natives into a proletariat by compelling them to work for wages in the colonies. It is responsible for the creation and expansion of spheres of interest for European capital in non-European regions, for extorting railway concessions in backward countries, and for enforcing the claims of European capital as international lender. Finally, militarism is a weapon in the competitive struggle between capitalist countries for areas of non-capitalist civilisation.

In addition, militarism has yet another important function. From the purely economic point of view, it is a pre-eminent means for the realisation of surplus value; it is in itself a province of accumulation. In examining the question who should

* Excerpts from Rosa Luxemburg, *The Accumulation of Capital* (New Haven: Yale University Press, 1951), pp. 454–7, 459 f., 464–7. [Originally published in 1913.]

count as a buyer for the mass of products containing the capitalised surplus value, we have again and again refused to consider the state and its organs as consumers. Since their income is derivative, they were all taken to belong to the special category of those who live on the surplus value (or partly on the wage of labour), together with the liberal professions and the various parasites of present-day society ('king, professor, prostitute, mercenary'). But this interpretation will only do on two assumptions: first, if we take it, in accordance with Marx's diagram, that the state has no other sources of taxation than capitalist surplus value and wages, and secondly, if we regard the state and its organs as consumers pure and simple. If the issue turns on the personal consumption of the state organs (as also of the 'mercenary') the point is that consumption is partly transferred from the working class to the hangers-on of the capitalist class, in so far as the workers foot the bill. . . .

With indirect taxation and high protective tariffs, the bill of militarism is footed mainly by the working class and the peasants. . . . The transfer of some of the purchasing power from the working class to the state entails a proportionate decrease in the consumption of means of subsistence by the working class. For capital as a whole, it means producing a smaller quantity of consumer goods for the working class, provided that both variable capital (in the form of money and as labour power) and the mass of appropriated surplus value remain constant, so that the workers get a smaller share of the aggregate product. . . . Capital has won with the left hand only what it has lost with the right. Or we might say that the large number of capitalists producing means of subsistence have lost the effective demand in favour of a small group of big armament manufacturers.

But this picture is only valid for individual capital. Here it makes no difference indeed whether production engages in one sphere of activity or another. As far as the individual capitalist is concerned, there are no departments of total production. . . . There are only commodities and buyers, and it is completely immaterial to him whether he produces instruments of life or instruments of death, corned beef or armour plating.

Opponents of militarism frequently appeal to this point of view to show that military supplies as an economic investment for capital merely put profit taken from one capitalist into the pocket of another. On the other hand, capital and its advocates try to overpersuade the working class to this point of view by talking them into the belief that indirect taxes and the demand of the state would only bring about a change in the material form of reproduction; instead of other commodities cruisers and guns would be produced which would give the workers as good a living, if not a better one. . . .

When we were formerly taking it for granted that the indirect taxes extorted from the workers are used for paying the officials and for provisioning the army, we found the 'saving' in the consumption of the working class to mean that the workers rather than the capitalists were made to pay for the personal consumption of the hangers-on of the capitalist class and the tools of their class-rule. This charge devolved from the surplus value to the variable capital, and a corresponding amount of the surplus value became available for purposes of capitalisation. Now we see how the taxes extorted from the workers afford capital a new opportunity for accumulation when they are used for armament manufacture.

On the basis of indirect taxation, militarism in practice works both ways. By lowering the normal standard of living for the working class, it ensures both that capital should be able to maintain a regular army, the organ of capitalist rule, and that it may tap an impressive field for further accumulation. . . .

Now the question arises, whether economic changes will result for capital, and if so, of what nature, from diverting the purchasing power of such strata to the state for militarist purposes. It almost looks as if we had come up against yet another shift in the material form of reproduction. Capital will now produce an equivalent of war materials for the state instead of producing large quantities of means of production and subsistence for peasant consumers. But in fact the changes go deeper. First and foremost, the state can use the mechanism of taxation to mobilise much larger amounts of purchasing power from the non-capitalist consumers than they would ordinarily spend on their own consumption. . . .

What would normally have been hoarded by the peasants

and the lower middle classes until it has grown big enough to invest in savings banks and other banks is now set free to constitute an effective demand and an opportunity for investment. Further the multitude of individual and insignificant demands for a whole range of commodities, which will become effective at different times and which might often be met just as well by simple commodity production, is now replaced by a comprehensive and homogeneous demand of the state. And the satisfaction of this demand presupposes a big industry of the highest order. It requires the most favourable conditions for the production of surplus value and for accumulation. In the form of government contracts for army supplies the scattered purchasing power of the consumers is concentrated in large quantities and, free of the vagaries and subjective fluctuations of personal consumption, it achieves an almost automatic regularity and rhythmic growth. Capital itself ultimately controls this automatic and rhythmic movement of militarist production through the legislature and a press whose function is to mould so-called 'public opinion'. That is why this particular province of capitalist accumulation at first seems capable of infinite expansion. All other attempts to expand markets and set up operational bases for capital largely depend on historical, social and political factors beyond the control of capital, whereas production for militarism represents a province whose regular and progressive expansion seems primarily determined by capital itself.

In this way capital turns historical necessity into a virtue: the ever fiercer competition in the capitalist world itself provides a field for accumulation of the first magnitude. Capital increasingly employs militarism for implementing a foreign and colonial policy to get hold of the means of production and labour power of non-capitalist countries and societies. This same militarism works in a like manner in the capitalist countries to divert purchasing power away from the non-capitalist strata. The representatives of simple commodity production and the working class are affected alike in this way. At their expense, the accumulation of capital is raised to the highest power, by robbing the one of their productive forces and by depressing the other's standard of living. Needless to say, after a certain stage the conditions for the accumulation of capital both at home and abroad turn into their very opposite—they become conditions for the decline of capitalism.

The more ruthlessly capital sets about the destruction of non-capitalist strata at home and in the outside world, the more it lowers the standard of living for the workers as a whole, the greater also is the change in the day-to-day history of capital. It becomes a string of political and social disasters and convulsions, and under these conditions, punctuated by periodical economic catastrophes or crises, accumulation can go on no longer.

*IIIA, 2. Bukharin, 'Capitalism and Armaments'**

When competition has finally reached its highest stage, when it has become competition between state capitalist trusts, then the use of state power, and the possibilities connected with it, begin to play a very large part.

The remnants of the old *laissez faire, laissez passer* ideology disappear, the epoch of the new 'mercantilism,' of imperialism, begins. . . .

If state power is generally growing in significance, the growth of its military organisation, the army and the navy, is particularly striking. The struggle between state capitalist trusts is decided in the first place by the relation between their military forces, for the military power of the country is the last resort of the struggling 'national' groups of capitalists. The immensely growing state budget devotes an ever larger share to 'defence purposes,' as militarisation is euphemistically termed.

The following table (see p. 154), illustrates the monstrous growth of military expenditues and their share in the state budget:

The present military budgets are expressed in the following figures: the United States (1914), $173,522,804 for the army and $139,682,186 for the navy, total $313,204,990; France (1913), 983,224,376 francs for the army and 467,176,109 francs for the navy, total 1,450,400,485 francs (in 1914, 1,717,202,233 francs); Russia (1913, counting only ordinary expenditures), 581,099,921 rubles for the army and

* Excerpts from N. Bukharin, *Imperialism and World Economy* (New York, 1929), pp. 123-7, 139 f., 170. [Originally published in 1915.]

244,846,500 rubles for the navy, total 825,946,421 rubles; Great Britain (1913–14), 28,220,000 pounds for the army and 48,809,300 pounds for the navy, total 77,029,300 pounds; Germany (1913, both ordinary and extraordinary expenditure), 97,845,960 pounds sterling, etc.

COST OF ARMY AND NAVY

States	*Years*	*Military expenditures per capita of the population*	*All state expenditures per capita of the population*	*Percentage of military expenditures in relation to all expenditures*	*Years*	*Military expenditures per capita of the population*	*All state expenditures per capita of the population*	*Percentage of military expenditures in relation to all expenditures*
England	1875	16.10	41.67	38.06	1907–08	26.42	54.83	48.6
France	1875	15.23	52.71	29.0	1908	24.81	67.04	37.0
Austria-Hungary	1873	5.92	22.05	26.8	1908	8.49	37.01	22.8
Italy	1874	6.02	31.44	19.1	1907–08	9.53	33.24	28.7
Russia	1877	5.24	15.14	34.6	1908	7.42	20.81	35.6
Japan	1875	0.60	3.48	17.2	1908	4.53	18.08	25.1
Germany	1881–2	9.43	33.07	28.5	1908	18.44	65.22	28.3
United States of America	1875	10.02	29.89	33.5	1907–08	16.68	29.32	56.9

We are now passing through a period when armaments on land, on water, and in the air are growing with feverish rapidity. Every improvement in military technique entails a reorganisation and reconstruction of the military mechanism; every innovation, every expansion of the military power of one state stimulates all the others. What we observe here is like the phenomenon we come across in the sphere of tariff policies where a raise of rates in one state is immediately reflected in all others, causing a general raise. Of course, here too, we have before us only a case of a general principle of competition, for the military power of the state capitalist trust is the weapon to be used in its economic struggle. The growth of armaments, creating as it does a demand for the products of the metallurgic industry, raises substantially the importance of heavy industry, particularly the importance of 'cannon kings' *à la* Krupp. To say, however, that wars are *caused* by the ammunition industry, would be a cheap assertion. The ammunition industry is by no means a branch of production existing for itself, it is not an artificially created evil which in turn calls forth the 'battle of nations.' It ought to be obvious from the foregoing considerations that armaments are an indispensable attribute of state power, an attribute that has a very definite function in the struggle among state capitalist trusts. Capitalist society is unthinkable without armaments, as it is unthinkable without wars. And just as it is true that not low prices cause competition but, on the contrary, competition causes low prices, it is equally true that not the existence of arms is the prime cause and the moving force in wars (although wars are obviously impossible without arms) but, on the contrary, the inevitableness of economic conflicts conditions the existence of arms. This is why in our times, when economic conflicts have reached an unusual degree of intensity, we are witnessing a mad orgy of armaments. Thus the rule of finance capital implies both imperialism and militarism. In this sense militarism is no less a typical historic phenomenon than finance capital itself....

But are not the costs of the struggle, *i.e.*, military expenditures, perchance so large that it does not pay for the bourgeoisie to continue in this way? Is not such a plan as the proposed militarisation of England an expression of bourgeois 'stupidity' which is blind to its own interests? Alas, it is not so. We must attribute this quality rather to the naïve pacifists than to the bourgeoisie. The latter keeps its balance sheet in perfect shape. The truth of the matter is that those who make such arguments ordinarily lose sight of all the complex functions of military power. Such power, as we have seen above, functions not only in times of war but also in times of peace, to back up its finance capital in 'peaceful competition.' The pacifists forget that the war burdens, due to the incidence of taxation, etc., are borne mainly by the working class, partly by the intermediary economic groupings which are being expropriated during the war (which means in the process of the greatest centralisation of production).

It follows from the above that the actual process of economic development will proceed in the midst of a sharpened struggle between the state capitalist trusts and the backward economic formations. A series of wars is unavoidable. In the historic process which we are to witness in the near future, world capitalism will move in the direction of a universal state capitalist trust by absorbing the weaker formations. Once the present war is over, new problems will have to be 'solved' by the sword. Partial agreements are, of course, possible here and there (*e.g.*, the fusion of Germany and Austria is quite probable). Every agreement or fusion, however, will only reproduce the bloody struggle on a new scale. Were 'Central Europe' to unite according to the plans of the German imperialists, the situation would remain comparatively the same; but even were *all* of Europe to unite, it would not yet signify 'disarmament.' It would signify an unheard of rise of militarism because the problem to be solved would be a colossal struggle between Europe on the one hand, America and Asia on the other. The struggle among small (small!) state capitalist trusts would be replaced by a struggle between still more colossal trusts. To attempt to eliminate this struggle by 'home remedies' and rose water is tantamount to bombarding an elephant with peas, for imperialism is not only a system most intimately connected with modern capitalism, it is also the most essential element of the latter. . . .

Capitalism has increased the power of militarism enormously. It has brought to the historic arena millions of armed men. The arms, however, begin to turn against capitalism itself. The masses of the people, aroused to political life and originally tame and docile, raise their voices ever higher. Steeled in battles forced upon them from above, accustomed to look into the face of death every minute, they begin to break the front of the imperialist war with the same fearlessness by turning it into civil war against the bourgeoisie. Thus capitalism, driving the concentration of production to extraordinary heights, and having created a centralised production apparatus, has therewith prepared the immense ranks of its own gravediggers. In the great clash of classes, the dictatorship of finance capital is being replaced by the dictatorship of the revolutionary proletariat. 'The hour of capitalist property has struck. The expropriators are being expropriated.'

*IIA, 3. Lenin, 'Imperialism and War'**

The principal feature of modern capitalism is the domination of monopolist combines of the big capitalists. These monopolies are most firmly established when *all* the sources of raw materials are controlled by the one group. And we have seen with what zeal the international capitalist combines exert every effort to make it impossible for their rivals to compete with them; for example, by buying up mineral lands, oil fields, etc. Colonial possession alone gives complete guarantee of success to the monopolies against all the risks of the struggle with competitors, including the risk that the latter will defend themselves by means of a law establishing a state monopoly. The more capitalism is developed, the more the need for raw materials is felt, the more bitter competition becomes, and the more feverishly the hunt for raw materials proceeds throughout the whole world, the more desperate becomes the struggle for the acquisition of colonies. . . .

Finance capital is not only interested in the already known sources of raw materials; it is also interested in potential sources of raw materials, because present-day technical development is extremely rapid, and because land which is useless today may be made fertile tomorrow if new methods are applied (to devise these new methods a big bank can equip a whole expedition of engineers, agricultural experts, etc.), and large amounts of capital are invested. This also applies to prospecting for minerals, to new methods of working up and utilising raw materials, etc., etc. Hence, the inevitable striving of finance capital to extend its economic territory and even its territory in general. In the same way that the trusts capitalise their property by estimating it at two or three times its value, taking into account its 'potential' (and not present) returns, and the further results of monopoly, so finance capital strives to seize the largest possible amount of land of all kinds and in any place it can, and by any means, counting on the possibilities of finding raw materials there, and fearing to be left behind in the insensate struggle for the last available

* Excerpts from V. I. Lenin, *Imperialism: The Highest Stage of Capitalism* (New York: International Publishers, 1939), pp. 82–5, 88 f., 97 f. [Originally published in 1917.]

scraps of undivided territory, or for the repartition of that which has been already divided. . . .

The necessity of exporting capital also gives an impetus to the conquest of colonies, for in the colonial market it is easier to eliminate competition, to make sure of orders, to strengthen the necessary 'connections,' etc., by monopolist methods (and sometimes it is the only possible way).

The non-economic superstructure which grows up on the basis of finance capital, its politics and its ideology, stimulates the striving for colonial conquest. 'Finance capital does not want liberty, it wants domination,' as Hilferding very truly says. . . .

Since we are speaking of colonial policy in the period of capitalist imperialism, it must be observed that finance capital and its corresponding foreign policy, which reduces itself to the struggle of the Great Powers for the economic and political division of the world, give rise to a number of *transitional* forms of national dependence. The division of the world into two main groups—of colony-owning countries on the one hand and colonies on the other—is not the only typical feature of this period; there is also a variety of forms of dependent countries; countries which, officially, are politically independent, but which are, in fact, enmeshed in the net of financial and diplomatic dependence. . . . Economically, the main thing in this process is the substitution of capitalist monopolies for capitalist free competition. Free competition is the fundamental attribute of capitalism, and of commodity production generally. Monopoly is exactly the opposite of free competition; but we have seen the latter being transformed into monopoly before our very eyes, creating large-scale industry and eliminating small industry, replacing large-scale industry by still larger-scale industry, finally leading to such a concentration of production and capital that monopoly has been and is the result: cartels, syndicates and trusts, and merging with them, the capital of a dozen or so banks manipulating thousands of millions. At the same time monopoly, which has grown out of free competition, does not abolish the latter, but exists over it and alongside of it, and thereby gives rise to a number of very acute, intense antagonisms, friction and higher conflicts. Monopoly is the transition from capitalism to a higher system.

If it were necessary to give the briefest possible definition of imperialism we should have to say that imperialism is the monopoly stage of capitalism. Such a definition would include what is most important, for, on the one hand, finance capital is the bank capital of a few big monopolist banks, merged with the capital of the monopolist combines of manufacturers; and, on the other hand, the division of the world is the transition from a colonial policy which has extended without hindrance to territories unoccupied by any capitalist power, to a colonial policy of monopolistic possession of the territory of the world which has been completely divided up. . . .

Imperialism is capitalism in that stage of development in which the dominance of monopolies and finance capital has established itself; in which the export of capital has acquired pronounced importance; in which the division of the world among the international trusts has begun; in which the division of all territories of the globe among the great capitalist powers has been completed. . . .

Finance capital and the trusts are increasing instead of diminishing the differences in the rate of development of the various parts of world economy. When the relation of forces is changed, how else, *under capitalism*, can the solution of contradictions be found, except by resorting to *violence*? . . .

Capitalism is growing with the greatest rapidity in the colonies and in overseas countries. Among the latter, *new* imperialist powers are emerging (*e.g.*, Japan). The struggle of world imperialism is becoming more acute. The tribute levied by finance capital on the most profitable colonial and overseas enterprises is increasing. In sharing out this 'booty,' an exceptionally large part goes to countries which, as far as the development of productive forces is concerned, do not always stand at the top of the list. In the case of the biggest countries, considered with their colonies, the total length of railways was as follows (in thousands of kilometres):

	1890	1913	Increase
U.S.A.	268	413	145
British Empire	107	208	101
Russia	32	78	46
Germany	43	68	25
France	41	63	22
Total	491	830	339

Thus, about 80 per cent of the total existing railways are concentrated in the hands of the five Great Powers. But the concentration of the *ownership* of these railways, of finance capital, is much greater still: French and English millionaires, for example, own an enormous amount of stocks and bonds in American, Russian and other railways.

Thanks to her colonies, Great Britain has increased the length of 'her' railways by 100,000 kilometres, four times as much as Germany. And yet, it is well known that the development of productive forces in Germany, and especially the development of the coal and iron industries, has been much more rapid during this period than in England—not to mention France and Russia. In 1892, Germany produced 4,900,000 tons of pig iron and Great Britain produced 6,800,000 tons; in 1912, Germany produced 17,600,000 tons and Great Britain 9,000,000 tons. Germany, therefore, had an overwhelming superiority over England in this respect. We ask, is there *under capitalism* any means of removing the disparity between the development of productive forces and the accumulation of capital on the one side, and the division of colonies and 'spheres of influence' for finance capital on the other side—other than by resorting to war?

*IIIA, 4. Mandel, 'Armaments and War Economy'**

Capitalism in decline is incapable of finding profitable use 'in a normal way' for the whole of the huge amount of capital it has accumulated. But capitalism cannot exist and grow without finding such profitable use, without constantly expanding its basis. In proportion as this structural crisis becomes more marked, the capitalist class, and especially the heads of the monopolies, more and more systematically seek out *replacement markets* which can guarantee such expansion. Armaments economy, war economy, represent the essential replacement markets which the capitalist system of production has found in its age of decline. . . .

The replacement market is, essentially a new purchasing-power created for the purchase of products of heavy industry by the state. But this purchasing-power is not 'created' in the

* Excerpts from Ernest Mandel, *Marxist Economic Theory* (London: Merlin Press, 1968), pp. 521-7.

literal sense of the word, that is, it does not spring from nowhere. It is not 'new', even when it appears in the form of bank notes freshly printed for this purpose by the state. Its only source is *a redistribution of the real national income*, a redistribution which can, of course, lead to an increase in production, that is in overall real income, which thus becomes an extra source of new purchasing power.

The shifting of purchasing power from one sector to another takes place through deductions made by the state, both direct and indirect, namely: direct taxes (on income, turnover, wealth, etc.); indirect taxes; more or less compulsory investment in state bonds; forced saving; printing of inflationary paper money which reduces the level of the workers' real wages, etc. It results in an enrichment of the heavy industrial monopolies at the expense of other strata of the population.

Thus, in the United States, of war contracts placed during the Second World War amounting to a total of 175 billion dollars, 67.2 per cent went to 100 monopoly trusts, mostly in heavy industry. In Germany between 1933 and September 1939 about 63 to 64 billion RM were spent on rearmament, which caused the production of capital goods (machinery and equipment) to increase fourfold as compared with 1932, while the production of consumer goods did not increase by so much as 50 per cent. During the Korean war, of all the war contracts placed between July 1950 and June 1953, the 100 biggest American firms received 64 per cent.

The role of replacement market played by the arms economy is indispensable for making possible profitable use of the capital of heavy industry and the 'overcapitalised' big monopolies. But the arms economy makes the state the chief customer of this industry. The special ties between the state and monopoly capital, which we have already stressed all through this analysis of the declining phase of capitalism, thus assume a more specific form.

The state, in close symbiosis with the monopolies, whose heads more and more often effect personal union with those who carry out key functions in the state machine, *guarantees the monopolies' profits not only by a policy of subsidies or insurance against loss, but also, and especially, by ensuring stable and permanent markets for them*: public contracts, which in the great majority of cases, are contracts for national defence. . . .

The ever-greater—and stable!—share of armament expenditure in the national income of all the capitalist nations is the chief factor determining the growth of 'public expenditure' in the national budget; the development of the social services plays only a secondary role in this connection—a role which often, moreover, is indirectly linked with the arms economy: thus, the social expenditure in the American budget of 1957–58 included 4.5 billion dollars for payments to ex-servicemen, etc. This public expenditure nowadays absorbs between 12 and 20 per cent of the gross national product of the chief capitalist countries. . . .

If war economy carried to its logical conclusion necessarily implies a process of contracted reproduction, this is not so with a more or less permanent economy of armaments and militarisation which is kept within certain limits. On the contrary: in this case the state's contracts stimulate production and expansion of productive capacity not only in the directly 'militarised' sectors, but also in the raw material sectors and even, through the increase in general demand thus created, in the consumer goods sectors. *So long as there are unused resources in society*, this 'stimulant' will tend to ensure full employment of them, while in the long run undermining the stability of the currency.

But as soon as full employment of means of production and labour has been achieved, no fresh expansion of military expenditure can take place without transfer of resources from other sectors of the economy to the militarised sectors (whether these transfers take place directly, by way of orders and decrees, or spontaneously, through the effect of price increases).

Even in this case, contracted reproduction does not necessarily set in in all sectors—it may be confined to certain sectors which are in direct competition with the arms sectors for the allocation of resources. Frequently, expanded reproduction may even continue in all sectors, on condition that the rate of expansion is stable or declining, that is, that the armaments sector absorbs the bulk or the whole of the *additional* resources available in the economy. . . .

Does this mean that a 'moderate' arms economy can guarantee full employment and give birth to a 'crisis-free capitalism'? Not at all. But before examining this problem we must draw attention to two other phenomena; the fact that the arms produced in order to secure a 'replacement market' for capitalism have the unfortunate tendency to be used, and the fact that the arms economy implies a permanent tendency to currency inflation.

The increasing role played by the arms economy, and by war economy in the strict sense, in making possible the profitable use of capital . . . becomes a subsidiary cause of imperialist wars and war dangers. The latter are phases which are more and more difficult to avoid in the production cycle of capitalism in its period of decline. To the extent that the armaments policy becomes a necessary palliative for crisis, or the threat of crisis, it produces its own inevitable prolongation in the threat of war. The extension of productive capacity which it entails intensifies still further the contradictions which it has striven to escape. A new and more dangerous day of reckoning approaches; the arms policy cannot be pursued indefinitely without the use-value of the accumulated weapons being exploited, that is, without the outbreak of wars, whether 'local' or general. The arms policy can follow a spiral course only in so far as the arms themselves are 'consumed', disappear, that is, in so far as war breaks out. Finally, technical progress threatens the accumulated weapons with a rapid 'moral depreciation'. All these factors create a pressure in the direction of war danger from the moment a certain point is reached in rearmament, war-preparation and rearmament acting on each other alternately as cause and effect.

The economic cycle is thus combined with a cycle of wars: this is the era of war capitalism. . . .

The creation of a permanent, and growing, armaments sector within the capitalist economy explains another typical phenomenon of the period of capitalist decline: the permanent tendency to currency inflation.

Indeed, arms production has, from the currency standpoint, this special feature: it increases the amount of purchasing power in circulation without creating on the market a corresponding additional supply of *goods*, as counter-value. Even when this increased purchasing power brings about the re-employment of previously idle machinery and men, it causes inflation eventually. The incomes of the workers and the profits of the companies reappear on the market as demand for consumer goods and capital goods, without the production of these goods having been increased.

There is only one special case where the production of armaments is not a cause of currency inflation, and that is when *all* arms expenditure has been financed *entirely by taxes* (that is, *by reducing the purchasing power* of individuals and firms) and when taxes do not change the rates between demand for consumer goods and demand for capital goods if the supply of these goods remains fixed. Such a case is practically unknown in the epoch of the decline of capitalism. . . .

IIIB. Socialism, Militarism, and Pacifism

1. The Position of Lenin on World War and Civil War

*a. Lenin, 'Socialism and War'** Socialists have always condemned wars between nations as barbarous and brutal. Our attitude towards war, however, is fundamentally different from that of the bourgeois pacifists (supporters and advocates of peace) and of the anarchists. We differ from the former in that we understand the inevitable connection between wars and the class struggle within a country; we understand that wars cannot be abolished unless classes are abolished and socialism is created; we also differ in that we regard civil wars, i.e., wars waged by an oppressed class against the oppressor class, by slaves against slaveholders, by serfs against landowners, and wage-workers against the bourgeoisie, as fully legitimate, progressive and necessary. We Marxists differ from both pacifists and anarchists in that we deem it necessary to study war historically (from the standpoint of Marx's dialectical materialism) and separately. There have been in the past numerous wars, which, despite all the horrors, atrocities, distress and suffering that inevitably accompany all wars, were progressive, i.e., benefited the development of mankind by helping to destroy most harmful and reactionary institutions

* Excerpts from V. I. Lenin, 'Socialism and War', *Collected Works*, xxi: 299-304, 308 f., 328 f., [Originally published in 1915.]

(e.g., an autocracy or serfdom) and the most barbarous despotisms in Europe (the Turkish and the Russian). That is why the features historically specific to the present war must come up for examination.

The Great French Revolution ushered in a new epoch in the history of mankind. From that time down to the Paris Commune, i.e., between 1789 and 1871, one type of war was of a bourgeois-progressive character, waged for national liberation. In other words, the overthrow of absolutism and feudalism, the undermining of these institutions, and the overthrow of alien oppression, formed the chief content and historical significance of such wars. These were therefore progressive wars; during *such* wars, all honest and revolutionary democrats, as well as all socialists, always wished success to that country (i.e., that bourgeoisie) which had helped to overthrow or undermine the most baneful foundations of feudalism, absolutism and the oppression of other nations. For example, the revolutionary wars waged by France contained an element of plunder and the conquest of foreign territory by the French, but this does not in the least alter the fundamental historical significance of those wars, which destroyed and shattered feudalism and absolutism in the whole of the old, serf-owning Europe. In the Franco-Prussian war, Germany plundered France but this does not alter the fundamental historical significance of that war, which liberated tens of millions of German people from feudal disunity and from the oppression of two despots, the Russian tsar and Napoleon III.

The period of 1789–1871 left behind it deep marks and revolutionary memories. There could be no development of the proletarian struggle for socialism prior to the overthrow of feudalism, absolutism and alien oppression. When, in speaking of the wars of *such* periods, socialists stressed the legitimacy of 'defensive' wars, they always had these aims in mind, namely revolution against medievalism and serfdom. By a 'defensive' war socialists have always understood a '*just*' war in this particular sense (Wilhelm Liebknecht once expressed himself precisely in this way). It is only in this sense that socialists have always regarded wars 'for the defence of the fatherland', or 'defensive' wars, as legitimate, progressive and just. For example, if tomorrow, Morocco were to declare war on France, or India on Britain, or Persia or China on Russia, and so on, these would be 'just', and 'defensive' wars, *irrespective* of who would be the first to attack; any socialist would wish the oppressed, dependent and unequal states victory over the oppressor, slaveholding and predatory 'Great' Powers.

But imagine a slave-holder who owns 100 slaves warring against another who owns 200 slaves, for a more 'just' redistribution of slaves. The use of the term of a 'defensive' war, or a war 'for the defence of the fatherland', would clearly be historically false in such a case and would in practice be sheer deception of the common people, philistines, and the ignorant, by the astute slave-holders. It is in this way that the peoples are being deceived with 'national' ideology and the term of 'defence of the fatherland', by the present-day imperialist bourgeoisie, in the war now being waged between slaveholders with the purpose of consolidating slavery.

It is almost universally admitted that this war is an imperialist war. In most cases, however, this term is distorted, or applied to one side, or else a loophole is left for the assertion that this war may, after all, be bourgeois-progressive, and of significance to the national-liberation movement. Imperialism is the highest stage in the development of capitalism, reached only in the twentieth century. Capitalism now finds that the old national states, without whose formation it could not have overthrown feudalism, are too cramped for it. Capitalism has developed concentration to such a degree that entire branches of industry are controlled by syndicates, trusts and associations of capitalist multimillionaires and almost the entire globe has been divided up among the 'lords of capital' either in the form of colonies, or by entangling other countries in thousands of threads of financial exploitation. Free trade and competition have been superseded by a striving towards monopolies, the seizure of territory for the investment of capital and as sources of raw materials, and so on. From the liberator of nations, which it was in the struggle against feudalism, capitalism in its imperialist stage has turned into the greatest oppressor of nations. Formerly progressive, capitalism has become reactionary; it has developed the forces of production to such a degree that mankind is faced with the alternative of adopting socialism or of experiencing years and even decades of armed struggle between the 'Great' Powers for the artificial preservation of capitalism by means of colonies, monopolies, privileges and national oppression of every kind. . . .

Since 1876, most of the nations which were foremost fighters for freedom in 1789-1871, have, on the basis of a highly developed and 'over-mature' capitalism, become oppressors and enslavers of most of the population and the nations of the globe. From 1876 to 1914, six 'Great' Powers grabbed 25 million square kilometres, i.e., an area two and half times that of Europe! Six Powers have enslaved *523 million* people in the colonies. For every four inhabitants in the 'Great' Powers there are five in 'their' colonies. It is common knowledge that colonies are conquered with fire and sword, that the population of the colonies are brutally treated, and that they are exploited in a thousand ways (by exporting capital, through concessions, etc., cheating in the sale of goods, submission to the authorities of the 'ruling' nation, and so on and so forth). The Anglo-French bourgeoisie are deceiving the people when they say that they are waging a war for the freedom of nations and of Belgium; in fact they are waging a war for the purpose of retaining the colonies they have grabbed and robbed. The German imperialists would free Belgium, etc., at once if the British and French would agree to 'fairly' share their colonies with them. A feature of the situation is that in this war the fate of the colonies is being decided by a war on the Continent. From the standpoint of bourgeois justice and national freedom (or the right of nations to existence), Germany might be considered absolutely in the right as against Britain and France, for she has been 'done out' of colonies, her enemies are oppressing an immeasurably far larger number of nations than she is, and the Slavs that are being oppressed by her ally, Austria, undoubtedly enjoy far more freedom than those of tsarist Russia, that veritable 'prison of nations'. Germany, however, is fighting, not for the liberation of nations, but for their oppression. It is not the business of socialists to help the younger and stronger robber (Germany) to plunder the older and overgorged robbers. Socialists must take advantage of the struggle between the robbers to overthrow all of them. To be able to do this, socialists must first of all tell the people the truth, namely, that this war is, in three respects, a war between slave-holders with the aim of consolidating slavery. This is a war, firstly, to increase the enslavement of the colonies by means of a 'more equitable' distribution and subsequent more concerted exploitation of them; secondly, to increase the oppression of other nations within the 'Great' Powers, since *both* Austria *and* Russia (Russia in greater degree and with results far worse than Austria) maintain their rule only by such oppression, intensifying it by means of war; and thirdly, to increase and prolong wage slavery, since the proletariat is split up and suppressed, while the capitalists are the gainers, making fortunes out of the war, fanning national prejudices and intensifying reaction, which has raised its head in all countries, even in the freest and most republican. . . .

The Russian social-chauvinists (headed by Plekhanov) make references to Marx's tactics in the war of 1870; the German (of the type of Lensch, David and Co.)—to Engels's statement in 1891 that, in the event of war against Russia and France combined, it would be the duty of the German socialists to defend their fatherland; finally, the social-chauvinists of the Kautsky type, who want to reconcile and legitimatise international chauvinism, refer to the fact that Marx and Engels, while condemning war, nevertheless, from 1854-55 to 1870-71 and 1876-77, always took the side of one belligerent state or another, once war had broken out.

All these references are outrageous distortions of the views of Marx and Engels, in the interest of the bourgeoisie and the opportunists, in just the same way as the writings of the anarchists Guillaume and Co. distort the views of Marx and Engels so as to justify anarchism. The war of 1870-71 was historically progressive on the part of Germany, until Napoleon III was defeated: the latter, together with the tsar, had oppressed Germany for years, keeping her in a state of feudal disunity. But as soon as the war developed into the plundering of France (the annexation of Alsace and Lorraine), Marx and Engels emphatically condemned the Germans. Even at the beginning of the war, Marx and Engels approved of the refusal of Bebel and Liebknecht to vote for war credits, and advised Social-Democrats not to merge with the bourgeoisie, but to uphold the independent class interests of the proletariat. To apply to the present imperialist war the appraisal of this bourgeois-progressive war of national liberation is a mockery of the truth. The same applies with still greater force to the war of 1854–55, and to all the wars of the nineteenth century, when there existed *no* modern imperialism, *no* mature objective conditions for socialism, and *no* mass socialist parties *in any* of the belligerent countries. . . .

Anyone who today refers to Marx's attitude towards the wars of the epoch of the *progressive* bourgeoisie, and forgets Marx's statement that 'the workingmen have no country'—a statement that applies *precisely* to the period of the reactionary and outmoded bourgeoisie, to the epoch of the socialist revolution, is shamelessly distorting Marx, and is substituting the bourgeois point of view for the socialist. . . . .

Conferences with so-called programmes of 'action' have till now confined themselves to announcing a more or less outspoken programme of sheer pacifism. Marxism is not pacifism. Of course, the speediest possible termination of the war must be striven for. However, the 'peace' demand acquires a proletarian significance only if a *revolutionary* struggle is called for. Without a series of revolutions, what is called a democratic peace is a philistine Utopia.

*IIIB, 1b. Lenin, 'The Military Program of the Proletarian Revolution'** Their principal argument is that the disarmament demand is the clearest, most decisive, most consistent expression of the struggle against all militarism and against all war.

But in this principal argument lies the disarmament advocates' principal error. Socialists cannot, without ceasing to be socialists, be opposed to all war.

Firstly, socialists have never been, nor can they ever be, opposed to revolutionary wars. The bourgeoisie of the imperialist 'Great' Powers has become thoroughly reactionary, and the war *this* bourgeoisie is now waging we regard as a reactionary, slave-owners' and criminal war. But what about a war *against* this bourgeoisie? A war, for instance, waged by peoples oppressed by and dependent upon this bourgeoisie, or by

* Excerpts from V. I. Lenin, 'The Military Program of the Proletarian Revolution', *Collected Works*, xxiii: 77–83, 85 f. [Originally published in 1916.]

colonial peoples, for liberation? In §5 of the *Internationale* group theses we read: 'National wars are no longer possible in the era of this unbridled imperialism.' That is obviously wrong.

The history of the twentieth century, this century of 'unbridled imperialism', is replete with colonial wars. But what we Europeans, the imperialist oppressors of the majority of the world's peoples, with our habitual, despicable European chauvinism, call 'colonial wars' are often national wars, or national rebellions of these oppressed peoples. One of the main features of imperialism is that it accelerates capitalist development in the most backward countries, and thereby extends and intensifies the struggle against national oppression. That is a fact, and from it inevitably follows that imperialism must often give rise to national wars. *Junius*, who defends the above-quoted 'theses' in her pamphlet, says that in the imperialist era every national war against an imperialist Great Power leads to the intervention of a rival imperialist Great Power. Every national war is thus turned into an imperialist war. But that argument is wrong too. This *can* happen, but does not always happen. Many colonial wars between 1900 and 1914 did not follow that course. And it would be simply ridiculous to declare, for instance, that after the present war, if it ends in the utter exhaustion of all the belligerents, 'there can be no' national, progressive, revolutionary wars 'of any kind', waged, say, by China in alliance with India, Persia, Siam, etc., against the Great Powers.

To deny all possibility of national wars under imperialism is wrong in theory, obviously mistaken historically, and tantamount to European chauvinism in practice: we who belong to nations that oppress hundreds of millions in Europe, Africa, Asia, etc., are invited to tell the oppressed peoples that it is 'impossible' for them to wage war against 'our' nations!

Secondly, civil war is just as much a war as any other. He who accepts the class struggle cannot fail to accept civil wars, which in every class society are the natural, and under certain conditions inevitable, continuation, development and intensification of the class struggle. That has been confirmed by every great revolution. To repudiate civil war, or to forget about it, is to fall into extreme opportunism and renounce the socialist revolution.

Thirdly, the victory of socialism in one country does not at one stroke eliminate all war in general. On the contrary, it presupposes wars. The development of capitalism proceeds extremely unevenly in different countries. It cannot be otherwise under commodity production. From this it follows irrefutably that socialism cannot achieve victory simultaneously *in all* countries. It will achieve victory first in one or several countries, while the others will for some time remain bourgeois or pre-bourgeois. This is bound to create not only friction, but a direct attempt on the part of the bourgeoisie of other countries to crush the socialist state's victorious proletariat. In such cases a war on our part would be a legitimate and just war. It would be a war for socialism, for the liberation of other nations from the bourgeoisie. Engels was perfectly right when, in his letter to Kautsky of September 12, 1882, he clearly stated that it was possible for *already victorious* socialism to wage 'defensive wars'. What he had in mind was defence of the victorious proletariat against the bourgeoisie of other countries.

Only after we have overthrown, finally vanquished and expropriated the bourgeoisie of the whole world, and not merely of one country, will wars become impossible. And from a scientific point of view it would be utterly wrong—and utterly unrevolutionary—for us to evade or gloss over the most important thing: crushing the resistance of the bourgeoisie—the most difficult task, and one demanding the greatest amount of fighting, in the *transition* to socialism. The 'social' parsons and opportunists are always ready to build dreams of future peaceful socialism. But the very thing that distinguishes them from revolutionary Social-Democrats is that they refuse to think about and reflect on the fierce class struggle and class *wars* needed to achieve that beautiful future.

We must not allow ourselves to be led astray by words. The term 'defence of the fatherland', for instance, is hateful to many because both avowed opportunists and Kautskyites use it to cover up and gloss over the bourgeois lie about the *present* predatory war. This is a fact. But it does not follow that we must no longer see through to the meaning of political slogans. To accept 'defence of the fatherland' in the present war is no more nor less than to accept it as a 'just' war, a war in the interests of the proletariat—no more nor less, we repeat, because invasions may occur in any war. It would be sheer folly to repudiate 'defence of the fatherland' *on the part* of oppressed nations in their wars *against* the imperialist Great Powers, or on the part of a victorious proletariat in *its* war against some Galliffet of a bourgeois state.

Theoretically, it would be absolutely wrong to forget that every war is but the continuation of policy by other means. The present imperialist war is the continuation of the imperialist policies of two groups of Great Powers, and these policies were engendered and fostered by the sum total of the relationships of the imperialist era. But this very era must also necessarily engender and foster policies of struggle against national oppression and of proletarian struggle against the bourgeoisie and, consequently, also the possibility and inevitability, first, of revolutionary national rebellions and wars; second, of proletarian wars and rebellions *against* the bourgeoisie; and, third, of a combination of both kinds of revolutionary war, etc.

To this must be added the following general consideration.

An oppressed class which does not strive to learn to use arms, to acquire arms, only deserves to be treated like slaves. We cannot, unless we have become bourgeois pacifists or opportunists, forget that we are living in a class society from which there is no way out, nor can there be, save through the class struggle. In every class society, whether based on slavery, serfdom, or, as at present, on wage-labour, the oppressor class is always armed. Not only the modern standing army, but even the modern militia—and even in the most democratic bourgeois republics, Switzerland, for instance—represent the bourgeoisie armed *against* the proletariat. That is such an elementary truth that it is hardly necessary to dwell upon it. Suffice it to point to the use of troops against strikers in all capitalist countries.

A bourgeoisie armed against the proletariat is one of the biggest, fundamental and cardinal facts of modern capitalist society. And in face of this fact, revolutionary Social-Democrats are urged to 'demand' 'disarmament'! That is tantamount to complete abandonment of the class-struggle point of view, to renunciation of all thought of revolution. Our slogan must be: arming of the proletariat to defeat, expropriate and disarm the bourgeoisie. These are the only tactics possible for a revolutionary class, tactics that follow logically from, and are dictated by, the whole *objective development* of capitalist militarism. Only *after* the proletariat has disarmed the bourgeoisie will it be able, without betraying its world-historic mission, to consign all armaments to the scrap-heap. And the proletariat will undoubtedly do this, but *only when this condition has been fulfilled, certainly not before.*

If the present war rouses among the reactionary Christian socialists, among the whimpering petty bourgeoisie, *only* horror and fright, only aversion to all use of arms, to bloodshed, death, etc., then we must say: Capitalist society is and has always been *horror without end.* If this most reactionary of all wars is now preparing for that society an *end in horror,* we have no reason to fall into despair. But the disarmament 'demand', or more correctly, the dream of disarmament, is, objectively, nothing but an expression of despair at a time when, as everyone can see, the bourgeoisie itself is paving the way for the only legitimate and revolutionary war—civil war against the imperialist bourgeoisie.

A lifeless theory, some might say, but we would remind them of two world-historical facts: the role of the trusts and the employment of women in industry, on the one hand, and the Paris Commune of 1871 and the December 1905 uprising in Russia, on the other.

The bourgeoisie makes it its business to promote trusts, drive women and children into the factories, subject them to corruption and suffering, condemn them to extreme poverty. We do not 'demand' such development, we do not 'support' it. We fight it. But *how* do we fight? We explain that trusts and the employment of women in industry are progressive. We do not want a return to the handicraft system, pre-monopoly capitalism, domestic drudgery for women. Forward through the trusts, etc., and beyond them to socialism!

With the necessary changes that argument is applicable also to the present militarisation of the population. Today the imperialist bourgeoisie militarises the youth as well as the adults; tomorrow, it may begin militarising the women. Our attitude should be: All the better! Full speed ahead! For the faster we move, the nearer shall we be to the armed uprising against capitalism. How can Social-Democrats give way to fear of the militarisation of the youth, etc., if they have not forgotten the example of the Paris Commune? This is not a 'lifeless theory' or a dream. It is a fact. And it would be a sorry state of affairs indeed if, all the economic and political facts notwithstanding, Social-Democrats began to doubt that the imperialist era and imperialist wars must inevitably bring about a repetition of such facts.

A certain bourgeois observer of the Paris Commune, writing to an English newspaper in May 1871, said: 'If the French nation consisted entirely of women, what a terrible nation it would be!' Women and teen-age children fought in the Paris Commune side by side with the men. It will be no different in the coming battles for the overthrow of the bourgeoisie. Proletarian women will not look on passively as poorly armed or unarmed workers are shot down by the well-armed forces of the bourgeoisie. They will take to arms, as they did in 1871, and from the cowed nations of today—or more correctly, from the present-day labour movement, disorganised more by the opportunists than by the governments—there will undoubtedly arise, sooner or later, but with absolute certainty, an international league of the 'terrible nations' of the revolutionary proletariat.

The whole of social life is now being militarised. Imperialism is a fierce struggle of the Great Powers for the division and redivision of the world. It is therefore bound to lead to further militarisation in all countries, even in neutral and small ones. How will proletarian women oppose this? Only by cursing all war and everything military, only by demanding disarmament? The women of an oppressed and really revolutionary class will never accept that shameful role. They will say to their sons: 'You will soon be grown up. You will be given a gun. Take it and learn the military art properly. The proletarians need this knowledge not to shoot your brothers, the workers of other countries, as is being done in the present war, and as the traitors to socialism are telling you to do. They need it to fight the bourgeoisie of their own country, to put an end to exploitation, poverty and war, and not by pious wishes, but by defeating and disarming the bourgeoisie.'

If we are to shun such propaganda, precisely such propaganda, in connection with the present war, then we had better stop using fine words about international revolutionary Social-Democracy, the socialist revolution and war against war. . . .

On the question of a militia, we should say: We are not in favour of a bourgeois militia; we are in favour only of a proletarian militia. Therefore, 'not a penny, not a man', not only for a standing army, but even for a bourgeois militia, even in countries like the United States, or Switzerland, Norway, etc. The more so that in the freest republican countries (e.g., Switzerland) we see that the militia is being increasingly Prussianised, particularly in 1907 and 1911, and prostituted by being used against strikers. We can demand popular election of officers, abolition of all military law, equal rights for foreign and native-born workers (a point particularly important for those imperialist states which, like Switzerland, are more and more blatantly exploiting larger numbers of foreign workers, while denying them all rights). Further, we can demand the right of every hundred, say, inhabitants of a given country to form voluntary military-training associations, with free election of instructors paid by the state, etc. Only under these conditions could the proletariat acquire military training for *itself* and not for its slave-owners; and the need for such training is imperatively dictated by the interests of the proletariat. The Russian revolution showed that every success of the revolutionary movement, even a partial success like the seizure of a certain city, a certain factory town, or winning over a certain section of the army, inevitably *compels* the victorious proletariat to carry out just such a programme. . . .

Disarmament as a social idea, i.e., an idea that springs from, and can affect, a certain social environment, and is not the invention of some crackpot, springs, evidently, from the peculiar 'tranquil' conditions prevailing, by way of exception, in certain small states, which have for a fairly long time stood aside from the world's path of war and bloodshed, and hope to remain that way. To be convinced of this, we have only to consider the arguments advanced, for instance, by the Norwegian advocates of disarmament. 'We are a small country,' they say. 'Our army is small; there is nothing we can do against the Great Powers [and, consequently, nothing we can do to resist forcible involvement in an imperialist *alliance* with one or the other Great-Power group]. . . . We want to be left in peace in our backwoods and continue our backwoods politics, demand disarmament, compulsory arbitration, permanent neutrality, etc.' ('permanent' after the Belgian fashion, no doubt?).

The petty striving of petty states to hold aloof, the petty-bourgeois desire to keep as far away as possible from the great battles of world history, to take advantage of one's relatively monopolistic position in order to remain in hidebound passivity—this is the *objective* social environment which may ensure the disarmament idea a certain degree of success and a certain degree of popularity in some of the small states. That striving is, of course, reactionary and is based entirely on illusions, for, in one way or another, imperialism draws the small states into the vortex of world economy and world politics.

*IIIB, 1c. Lenin, '"Left-Wing" Childishness and the Petty-Bourgeois Mentality'** It is because you devote more effort to learning by heart and committing to memory revolutionary slogans than to thinking them out. This leads you to write 'the defence of the socialist fatherland' in quotation marks, which are probably meant to signify your attempts at being ironical, but which really prove that you are muddleheads. You are accustomed to regard 'defencism' as something base and despicable; you have learned this and committed it to memory. You have learned this by heart so thoroughly that some of you have begun talking nonsense to the effect that defence of the fatherland in an imperialist *epoch* is impermissible (as a matter of fact, it is impermissible only in an imperialist, reactionary war, waged by the bourgeoisie). But you have not thought out why and when 'defencism' is abominable.

To recognise defence of the fatherland means recognising the legitimacy and justice of war. Legitimacy and justice from what point of view? Only from the point of view of the socialist proletariat and its struggle for its emancipation. We do not recognise any other point of view. If war is waged by the

* Excerpts from V. I. Lenin, '"Left-Wing" Childishness and the Petty-Bourgeois Mentality', *Collected Works*, xxvii: 331-3. [Originally published in 1920.]

exploiting class with the object of strengthening its rule as a class, such a war is a criminal war, and 'defencism' in *such* a war is a base betrayal of socialism. If war is waged by the proletariat after it has conquered the bourgeoisie in its own country, and is waged with the object of strengthening and developing socialism, such a war is legitimate and 'holy'.

We have been 'defencists' since October 25, 1917. I have said this more than once very definitely, and you dare not deny this. It is precisely in the interests of 'strengthening the connection' with international socialism that we *are in duty bound* to defend our *socialist* fatherland. Those who treat frivolously the defence of the country in which the proletariat has already achieved victory are the ones who destroy the connection with international socialism. When we were the representatives of an oppressed class we did not adopt a frivolous attitude towards defence of the fatherland in an imperialist war. We opposed such defence on principle. Now that we have become representatives of the ruling class, which has begun to organise socialism, we demand that everybody adopt a *serious* attitude towards defence of the country. And adopting a serious attitude towards defence of the country means thoroughly preparing for it, and strictly calculating the balance of forces. If our forces are obviously small, the best means of defence is *retreat into the interior of the country* (anyone who regards this as an artificial formula, made up to suit the needs of the moment, should read old Clausewitz, one of the greatest authorities on military matters, concerning the lessons of history to be learned in this connection). The 'Left Communists', however, do not give the slightest indication that they understand the significance of the question of the balance of forces.

When we were opposed to defencism on principle we were justified in holding up to ridicule those who wanted to 'save' their fatherland, ostensibly in the interests of socialism. When we gained the right to be proletarian defencists the whole question was radically altered. It has become our duty to calculate with the utmost accuracy the different forces involved, to weigh with the utmost care the chances of our ally (the international proletariat) being able to come to our aid in time. It is in the interest of capital to destroy its enemy (the revolutionary proletariat) bit by bit, before the workers in all countries have united (actually united, i.e., by beginning the revolution). It is in our interest to do all that is possible, to take advantage of the slightest opportunity to postpone the decisive battle until the moment (or *until after* the moment) the revolutionary workers' contingents have united in a single great international army.

IIIB, 2. Mao Tse-tung on War

*a. Mao, 'The Aim of War is to Eliminate War'** War, this monster of mutual slaughter among men, will be finally eliminated by the progress of human society, and in the not too distant future too. But there is only one way to eliminate it and that is to oppose war with war, to oppose counter-revolutionary war with revolutionary war, to oppose national counter-revolutionary war with national revolutionary war, and to oppose counter-revolutionary class war with revolutionary class war. History knows only two kinds of war, just and unjust. We support just wars and oppose unjust wars. All counter-revolutionary wars are unjust, all revolutionary wars are just. Mankind's era of wars will be brought to an end by our own efforts, and beyond doubt the war we wage is part of the final battle. But also beyond doubt the war we face will be part of the biggest and most ruthless of all wars. The biggest and most ruthless of unjust counter-revolutionary wars is hanging over us, and the vast majority of mankind will be ravaged unless we raise the banner of a just war. The banner of mankind's just war is the banner of mankind's salvation. The banner of China's just war is the banner of China's salvation. A war waged by the great majority of mankind and of the Chinese people is beyond doubt a just war, a most lofty and glorious undertaking for the salvation of mankind and China, and a bridge to a new era in world history. When human society advances to the point where classes and states are eliminated, there will be no more wars, counter-revolutionary or revolutionary, unjust or just; that will be the era of perpetual peace for mankind. Our study of the laws of

* Excerpts from Mao Tse-tung, 'Problems of Strategy in China's Revolutionary War' (Dec. 1936), *Selected Military Writings*, pp. 80 f.

revolutionary war springs from the desire to eliminate all wars; herein lies the distinction between us Communists and all the exploiting classes.

*IIIB, 2b. Mao, 'Fighting for Perpetual Peace'**

The protracted nature of China's anti-Japanese war is inseparably connected with the fight for perpetual peace in China and the whole world. Never has there been a historical period such as the present in which war is so close to perpetual peace. For several thousand years since the emergence of classes, the life of mankind has been full of wars; each nation has fought countless wars, either internally or with other nations. In the imperialist epoch of capitalist society, wars are waged on a particularly extensive scale and with a peculiar ruthlessness. The first great imperialist war of twenty years ago was the first of its kind in history, but not the last. Only the war which has now begun comes close to being the final war, that is, comes close to the perpetual peace of mankind. . . .

There will be no interruption in the development of the present war into a world war; mankind will not be able to avoid the calamity of war. Why then do we say the present war is near to perpetual peace? The present war is the result of the development of the general crisis of world capitalism which began with World War I; this general crisis is driving the capitalist countries into a new war and, above all, driving the fascist countries into new war adventures. This war, we can foresee, will not save capitalism, but will hasten its collapse. It will be greater in scale and more ruthless than the war of twenty years ago, all nations will inevitably be drawn in, it will drag on for a very long time, and mankind will suffer greatly. But, owing to the existence of the Soviet Union and the growing political consciousness of the people of the world, great revolutionary wars will undoubtedly emerge from this war to oppose all counter-revolutionary wars, thus giving this war the character of a struggle for perpetual peace. Even if later there should be another period of war, perpetual world peace will not be far off. Once man has eliminated capitalism, he will attain the era of perpetual peace, and there will be no

* Excerpts from Mao Tse-tung, 'On Protracted War' (May 1938), *Selected Military Writings*, pp. 222 ff.

more need for war. Neither armies, nor warships, nor military aircraft, nor poison gas will then be needed. Thereafter and for all time, mankind will never again know war. The revolutionary wars which have already begun are part of the war for perpetual peace. The war between China and Japan, two countries which have a combined population of over 500 million, will take an important place in this war for perpetual peace, and out of it will come the liberation of the Chinese nation. The liberated new China of the future will be inseparable from the liberated new world of the future. Hence our War of Resistance Against Japan takes on the character of a struggle for perpetual peace.

History shows that wars are divided into two kinds, just and unjust. All wars that are progressive are just, and all wars that impede progress are unjust. We Communists oppose all unjust wars that impede progress, but we do not oppose progressive, just wars. Not only do we Communists not oppose just wars, we actively participate in them. As for unjust wars, World War I is an instance in which both sides fought for imperialist interests; therefore the Communists of the whole world firmly opposed that war. The way to oppose a war of this kind is to do everything possible to prevent it before it breaks out and, once it breaks out, to oppose war with war, to oppose unjust war with just war, whenever possible. Japan's war is an unjust war that impedes progress, and the peoples of the world, including the Japanese people, should oppose it and are opposing it. In our country the people and the government, the Communist Party and the Kuomintang, have all raised the banner of righteousness in the national revolutionary war against aggression. Our war is sacred and just, it is progressive and its aim is peace. The aim is peace not just in one country but throughout the world, not just temporary but perpetual peace.

*IIIB, 3. Byely, 'Social and Political Character of Contemporary War'**

The history of class society abounds in military clashes and conflicts. In the past 5,500 years mankind was plunged into

* Excerpts from Byely *et al., Marxism–Leninism on War and Army* (1972), pp. 13 ff., 24 f., 48, 50 ff., 87, 194 f.

war more than 14,000 times. In the first half of this century alone there were two destructive world wars. All social progress in antagonistic formations brings bloodshed and suffering to the people. In the words of Marx, this progress was like a 'hideous pagan idol, who would not drink the nectar but from the skulls of the slain'.

But, wars are no fatal inevitability in human social development, they are a socio-historical phenomenon. There was a time when people did not know wars, and a time will come when wars will have been done away with once and for all.

As all socio-historical phenomena, the emergence of wars, their nature and place in history are subject to the laws of social development revealed by Marxism–Leninism. . . .

In class society war has become a means of resolving the antagonistic contradictions of social development.

The armed clashes between primeval tribes were a sideline occupation, an aspect of the labour process, admittedly a unique one, directed at the seizure of hunting grounds, pastures, etc. Marx characterised the armed struggle of primeval tribes as a great *common effort*, directed at the solution of the common task of seizing objective subsistence conditions, at their preservation and protection. All the male members of the tribal group, sometimes also the women, had to participate in this 'war'. All able-bodied members participated in 'combat' with their instruments of labour, their hunting weapons, since at that time these were the only instruments used in the struggle for existence. Armed clashes often ended in the destruction of some tribes, but never in their enslavement. Prisoners were not made slaves. They were either eaten, or became fully-fledged members of the victorious tribe. At that stage there were as yet no social forces to organise and conduct wars so as to achieve definite economic and political aims. There were also no special organisation of armed people, as there were no special arms for fighting.

Hence, *the armed clashes of primeval tribal groups and clans, who did not know private ownership and division into classes, were not wars in the real sense of the word.*

The point is that war has two organically interrelated aspects—the socio-political and the military-technical. The first expresses the social, class nature of war, its political essence; the second characterises the specifics of the war, of the armed struggle. In using the term 'war' to designate armed clashes in pre-class society, Marx and Engels referred to the second aspect. Clashes between tribes are reminiscent of wars in exploiter societies only by their second aspect.

War emerged as a socio-political phenomenon at a definite stage of social development, namely, with the disintegration of the primeval system and the emergence of the slave-owning mode of production, when private ownership of the means of production appeared, when society was divided into antagonistic classes, and the state emerged. Private property bred social violence. The exploiter classes legalised organised armed struggle aimed at winning material gains, enslaving people and enhancing the economic and political rule of those classes.

Exposing the vulgar 'force theory', Engels showed that it was not war that had given rise to property inequality and classes, but, on the contrary, that private ownership and the division of society into classes had transformed the armed clashes of primeval tribes into war as a socio-political phenomenon. Only then did wars become a constant venture of the exploiters.

Thus, *as a socio-historical phenomenon, serving the political aims of definite classes, war first emerged in exploiter society; it is the product and constant concomitant of class antagonistic society. . . .*

Wars, as we have shown above, are rooted in the nature of class-antagonistic formations. As distinct from crises of overproduction, that shake the capitalist economy periodically, wars do not emerge spontaneously. Crises are neither planned nor organised, nobody wants them or strives after them. They befall people spontaneously, like unavoidable natural calamities.

Wars unleashed by aggressive states are generally caused by various spontaneous processes, which assume so vast a scale that the countries concerned could neither foresee nor prevent them (financial crises and bankruptcies, uneven development of individual countries in economic respects and in world trade, rapid growth of the dissatisfaction of the people and adoption by them of revolutionary attitudes, etc.). The results of these wars generally differ from the aims for which they were unleashed and are sometimes directly opposed to them. This was characteristic of the last two world wars.

Yet, wars were the most organised and purposeful undertakings spontaneously developing societies ever carried out. Wars always demanded the overcoming to the maximum of social disorganisation and the suppression of spontaneity in the actions of large masses of people, and the subordination of these actions to a single guiding will. Generally, aggressive wars of the exploiter classes are prepared in secret conclave, but they are prepared deliberately and systematically over decades, and are unleashed just as deliberately by their governments and parties, at a moment considered by them most opportune and suitable for the beginning of the long-premeditated war. These parties, state bodies and leaders are the instigators of the war, and the responsibility for it lies with them.

Thus, *wars emerge neither spontaneously nor automatically. They are deliberately prepared and unleashed by definite parties and governments of the imperialist states. . . .*

Capitalism created a world market for the first time in history and enlarged the number of objects over which wars were waged. Chief among them were colonies—sources of cheap raw materials and labour power, spheres for the export of goods and capital, strongholds on international trade routes. For several centuries bourgeois Holland, Britain, France, Portugal and other European states waged wars of conquest against the weakly developed countries in order to make colonies of them. There were also wars between the capitalist countries themselves for a division of the world. . . .

Uneven development inevitably leads to abrupt changes in the alignment of forces in the world capitalist system. From time to time a sharp disturbance of the equilibrium occurs within that system. The old distribution of spheres of influence among the monopolies clashes with the new alignment of forces in the world. To bring the distribution of colonies in accord with the new balance of forces, there inevitably have to be periodical redivisions of the already divided world. Under capitalism armed violence is the only way of dividing up colonies and spheres of influence. . . .

As a result of the social antagonisms inherent in capitalism and the operation of the law of the uneven, leap-like economic and political development of the capitalist countries under imperialism, the contradictions between the bourgeois states aggravate to the utmost, and this leads to a division of the capitalist world into hostile coalitions, and to wars between them. . . .

However, the main contradiction now is that between the two opposing social systems—capitalism and socialism.

The contradictions between the two world systems are class contradictions. The socialist system greatly diminishes the sphere of imperialist exploitation and domination, creating conditions in which capitalism will lose the privileges it still enjoys. Socialism has a revolutionising influence on the working people in the capitalist countries, the colonies and dependent countries.

Another reason for the growing aggressiveness of modern imperialism is that the contradictions between the imperialist states, on the one hand, and the colonies and recent colonies, on the other, have greatly aggravated. . . .

The third cause is the exacerbation of the internal contradictions of capitalism after the Second World War. This is linked, first and foremost, with the continuing aggravation and deepening of the general crisis of capitalism, with the fact that the main contradiction of capitalist society, that between labour and capital, continues to grow. The transition from monopoly capitalism to state monopoly capitalism, under which the monopolies merge with the state, intensifies the exploitation of the working people, makes science and technology and the growing productive forces serve the aim of enriching a handful of monopolists. Exploitation has never been as hideous as it is today. Even when business conditions are favourable millions of people, workers and intellectuals are unemployed, and peasants are ruined and evicted from their land. At the same time a small number of powerful monopolies is profiting from the exploitation of the working people, from the arms race and aggressive wars.

State monopoly capitalism is responsible for the unprecedented intensification of militarism, including the economic and ideological fields. Militarisation permeates the entire life of bourgeois society. The production of mass-destruction weapons eats up an enormous part of the national income of the bourgeois states. During the past 20 years US military spending has increased more than 48-fold over that in the two prewar decades. More than 75 per cent of the total expenditure in the US Federal Budget is directly or indirectly channeled to military needs. The growth in weapons production in the main imperialist states makes other countries spend large funds on strengthening their defence too.

The imperialist state is becoming a militaristic police state. The economic superstructure rising on the basis of finance capital, and the politics and ideology of the finance oligarchy strengthen the state's aggressiveness. Under state-monopoly capitalism 'big business', the political leaders and the top brass controlling the state, make it pursue a policy aimed at preparing a war against the Soviet Union and other socialist states.

The sharp diminution of the sphere of action of the imperialist forces and the extreme aggravation of the contradictions under state-monopoly capitalism make the economic and political development of the bourgeois countries ever more uneven. This is the fourth reason responsible for the greater aggressiveness of the imperialist states. . . .

Just wars are distinguished from unjust ones by the progressive or reactionary, liberating or aggressive aims of the belligerents.

Any war that is waged by a people for the sake of freedom and social progress, for liberation from exploitation and national oppression or in defence of its state sovereignty, against an aggressive attack, is a just war.

Conversely, any war unleashed by the imperialists with the aim of seizing foreign territories, enslaving and plundering other peoples, is an unjust war. Such wars, continuing the policies of the imperialist bourgeoisie, are aimed at holding back by violence the logical course of social development, to suppress the revolutionary-liberation movements of the oppressed classes and peoples, and to strengthen the exploiter system. . . .

The First and Second World Wars hastened the coalescence of the capitalist monopolies with the bourgeois state, while state-monopoly capitalism led to a further intensification of militarism. A close union has formed between the army big brass and monopoly capital, and between monopoly capital and the top leaders of the state. State leadership has increasingly fallen under the influence of reactionary generals and monopolies in war production. The state has become a committee for managing the affairs of the monopoly bourgeoisie, the armed forces—a weapon for the implementation of their imperialist politics.

IIIC. Marxism–Leninism, the Army, and the Dictatorship of the Proletariat

*1. Lenin, 'The Function of the Army'**

One of the principal premises advanced, although not always definitely expressed, in favour of disarmament is this: we are opposed to war, to all war in general, and the demand for disarmament is the most definite, clear and unambiguous expression of this point of view.

We showed the fallacy of that idea in our review of Junius's pamphlet, to which we refer the reader. Socialists cannot be opposed to all war in general without ceasing to be socialists. We must not allow ourselves to be blinded by the present imperialist war. Such wars between 'Great' Powers are typical of the imperialist epoch; but democratic wars and rebellions, for instance, of oppressed nations against their oppressors to free themselves from oppression, are by no means impossible. Civil wars of the proletariat against the bourgeoisie for socialism are inevitable. Wars are possible between one country in which socialism has been victorious and other, bourgeois or reactionary, countries.

Disarmament is the ideal of socialism. There will be no wars in socialist society; consequently, disarmament will be achieved. But whoever expects that socialism will be achieved *without* a social revolution and the dictatorship of the proletariat is not a socialist. Dictatorship is state power based directly on *violence.* And in the twentieth century—as in the age of civilisation generally—violence means neither a fist nor a club, but *troops.* To put 'disarmament' in the programme is tantamount to making the general declaration: We are opposed to the use

* Excerpts from V. I. Lenin, 'The Disarmament Slogan' (1916), *Collected Works*, xxiii: 95.

of arms. There is as little Marxism in this as there would be if we were to say: We are opposed to violence!

IIIC, 2. Trotsky on the Discipline and Function of the Army

*a. Trotsky, 'Discipline of Army'** At this point I must say that those comrades who spoke here in the name of a new military doctrine have completely failed to convince me. I see in it a most dangerous thing: 'We'll crush our enemies beneath a barrage of red caps.' This happens to be ancient Russian doctrine.

As a matter of fact, what did some comrades say? They said that our doctrine consists not in commanding but in persuading, convincing and impressing through authoritativeness. A wonderful idea! The best thing would be to give Comrade Lyamin 3,000 Tambov deserters and let him organize a regiment with his method. I would very much like to see it done. But how is it possible to do anything at all by a mere stroke of the pen in the face of differences in cultural levels and in the face of ignorance? Our regime is called a regime of dictatorship; we do not conceal this. But some people say that what we need are not commanders-in-chief but commanders-in-persuasion. That's what Kerensky had.

Authoritativeness is an excellent thing, but not very tangible. If one were to impress solely through authoritativeness than what need have we for the *Cheka* and the Special Department? Finally, if we can impress a Tambov moujik solely through our authoritativeness, then why shouldn't we do the same with regard to the German and French peasants?

Comrade Vatsetis reminded us that truth is mightier than force. That is not so. What is correct is only this, that those oppressors who were ashamed of the brute force they applied always covered it up with hypocrisy. Truth is not superior to force; it cannot withstand the onset of artillery. Against artillery only artillery is effective. If you say that the cultural level of peasants and moujiks must be raised, then you are uttering what is an old truth to us. We are all for it and our state apparatus and, in particular, our military affairs must proceed along this line. But it is naive to think that such a task can be solved on the morrow. . . .

* Excerpts from L. Trotsky, 'Unified Military Doctrine' (Nov. 1921), *Military Writings*, pp. 24, 28 f.

And now, Comrades, I sum up briefly. He speaks the truth who says with regard to the will to victory that the ability is not always to be observed among our commanding staff to develop partial victories and partial successes to full victory. An explanation for this is to be found in the worker-peasant composition of our new commanding staff which inclines to be very easily satisfied with the very first successes attained. . . .

It is necessary to instill in the minds of our platoon, battalion and division commanders that they must possess not only the will to victory but must also know how to make reports and understand the meaning of maintaining communications, setting up guards, gathering intelligence. And for this the experience of old practice must be utilized. We must study our ABC's. Of no earthly use to us is a military doctrine that declares: 'We'll crush our enemies beneath a barrage of red caps.' We must eradicate such bravado and revolutionary snobbery. Chaos results whenever strategy is developed from the standpoint of revolutionary youth. Why? Because they have not learned the statutes thoroughly. We looked upon the Czarist statutes with disdain, and thanks to this did not teach them. Yet the old statutes prepare the new.

Marxists have always assimilated the old knowledge; they studied Feuerbach, Hegel, the French encyclopedists and materialists, and political economy. Marx devoted himself to the study of higher mathematics after his hair had grown grey. Engels studied military affairs and natural sciences. It will do incalculable harm if we were to inoculate the military youth with the idea that the old doctrine is utterly worthless and that we have entered a new epoch when everything can be viewed superciliously and with the equipment of an ignoramus. . . .

Meanwhile, let us not tear ourselves away from elementary needs, rations and boots. I think that a good ration is superior to a poor doctrine; and as touches boots, I maintain that our military doctrine begins with this, that we must tell the Red Army soldier: Learn to grease your boots, and oil your rifle. If in addition to our will to victory and our readiness to self-sacrifice we also learn to grease boots, then we shall have the best possible military doctrine.

*IIIC, 2b. Trotsky, 'Function of Army'** Marxism does not supply ready-made prescriptions, least of all in the sphere of military construction. But here, too, it provided us with the method. For if it is correct that war is a continuation of politics by other means, then it follows that the army, with bayonets held ready, is the continuation and the capstone of the entire social-state structure. . . .

The Red Army is the military expression of the proletarian dictatorship. Those who require a more solemn formula might say that the Red Army is the military embodiment of the 'doctrine' of proletarian dictatorship; in the first place, because the proletarian dictatorship is rendered secure by the Red Army; secondly, because the dictatorship of the proletariat would be impossible without the Red Army.

The misfortune, however, lies in this, that the awakening of military-theoretical interests engendered in the beginning a revival of certain doctrinaire prejudices of the first period of building the Red Army—prejudices which, to be sure, have been invested with certain new formulations, but nowise improved thereby. Certain perspicacious innovators have suddenly discoverd that *we are living, or rather not living at all but simply vegetating without military doctrine*, just like the king in Anderson's fairy tale who used to go naked without knowing it. There are some who say: 'It is high time we created the doctrine of the Red Army.' Others sing in chorus: 'We haven't been able to find the correct road on all practical questions of military construction for the lack of answers up to the present time to such fundamental questions of military doctrine as: What is the Red Army? What are the historical tasks before us? Will the Red Army have to wage defensive or offensive revolutionary wars? And so on and so forth.'

From the way things are put, it turns out that we were able to create the Red Army and, furthermore, a victorious Red Army, but, you see, we failed to supply it with a military doctrine. And this Red Army continues to thrive unregenerate. To the point-blank question of what the doctrine of the Red Army should be, we get the following answer: It must comprise the sum total of the elementary principles of building,

* Excerpts from L. Trotsky, 'Military Doctrine or Pseudo-Military Doctrinairism' (1921), *Military Writings*, pp. 34, 36 f.

educating and applying our armed forces. But this is a purely formal answer. The existing Red Army, too, has its own principles of 'building, educating and applying.' But under discussion is what kind of doctrine *are we lacking?* That is, what are these *new* principles, which must enter into the program of military construction, and just what is their content? And it is precisely here that the most incredible kind of muddling begins. One individual makes the sensational discovery that the Red Army is a *class* army, the army of proletarian dictatorship. Another one adds to this that inasmuch as the Red Army is a revolutionary, internationalist army, it must be an offensive army. A third proposes in behalf of the spirit of the offensive that we pay special attention to cavalry and aviation. And, finally, a fourth proposes that we don't forget to apply Makhno's hand carts. Around the world in a hand cart—there is a doctrine for the Red Army! It must be said, however, that in all these discoveries any kernel of healthy, not new but correct, ideas is absolutely lost in the husk of idle chatter.

*IIIC, 3. Mao, 'The Role of the Army'**

In other countries there is no need for each of the bourgeois parties to have an armed force under its direct command. But things are different in China, where, because of the feudal division of the country, those landlord or bourgeois groupings or parties which have guns have power, and those which have more guns have more power. Placed in such an environment, the party of the proletariat should see clearly to the heart of the matter.

Communists do not fight for personal military power (they must in no circumstances do that, and let no one ever again follow the example of Chang Kuo-tao), but they must fight for military power for the Party, for military power for the people. As a national war of resistance is going on, we must also fight for military power for the nation. Where there is naivety on the question of military power, nothing whatsoever can be achieved. It is very difficult for the labouring people, who have been deceived and intimidated by the reac-

* Excerpts from Mao Tse-tung, 'Problems of War and Strategy' (Nov. 6, 1938), *Selected Military Writings*, pp. 274 f.

tionary ruling classes for thousands of years, to awaken to the importance of having guns in their own hands. Now that Japanese imperialist oppression and the nation-wide resistance to it have pushed our labouring people into the arena of war, Communists should prove themselves the most politically conscious leaders in this war. Every Communist must grasp the truth, 'Political power grows out of the barrel of a gun.' Our principle is that the Party commands the gun, and the gun must never be allowed to command the Party. Yet, having guns, we can create Party organizations, as witness the powerful Party organizations which the Eighth Route Army has created in northern China. We can also create cadres, create schools, create culture, create mass movements. Everything in Yenan has been created by having guns. All things grow out of the barrel of a gun. According to the Marxist theory of the state, the army is the chief component of state power. Whoever wants to seize and retain state power must have a strong army. Some people ridicule us as advocates of the 'omnipotence of war'. Yes, we are advocates of the omnipotence of revolutionary war; that is good, not bad, it is Marxist. The guns of the Russian Communist Party created socialism. We shall create a democratic republic. Experience in the class struggle in the era of imperialism teaches us that it is only by the power of the gun that the working class and the labouring masses can defeat the armed bourgeoisie and landlords; in this sense we may say that only with guns can the whole world be transformed. We are advocates of the abolition of war, we do not want war; but war can only be abolished through war, and in order to get rid of the gun it is necessary to take up the gun.

*IIIC, 4. Byely, 'Structure, Discipline and Function of Army under Socialism'**

The laws governing the proletariat's class struggle against the bourgeoisie require that the socialist state should form armed forces. It is compelled to do so by the exploiter classes. The latter are the first to resort to armed violence against the working people. Therefore, in order to consolidate their power,

* Excerpts from Byely *et al.*, *Marxism–Leninism on War and Army* (1972), pp. 218–21, 238–40, 245 f., 248, 345.

to uphold their revolutionary gains and to defend the socialist country, the working class has to create powerful armed forces. 'If the ruling class, the proletariat,' Lenin said, 'wants to hold power, it must, therefore, prove its ability to do so by its military organisation.'

In the transition period from capitalism to socialism, especially immediately after the seizure of power by the proletariat, world imperialist reaction endeavours to stifle the socialist revolution by force. It supports and directs the resistance of internal counter-revolutionaries, organises armed actions against the power of the workers and peasants and supports counter-revolutionary troops when foreign interventionists invade the country. The function of armed defence of the socialist country against attacks from the outside, one of the basic functions of the workers' and peasants' state, merges with the function of suppressing armed resistance of the overthrown exploiters.

This function could have been carried out successfully by the socialist militia, if the internal counter-revolutionaries had not been helped by the armed forces of the imperialist powers. But the alliance of external and internal reaction for the purpose of restoring capitalism in the country makes it necessary to set up a regular, standing army. It has the functions of suppressing the armed resistance of the overthrown exploiter classes and of defending the country against the military attacks of international imperialism.

Externally the first function resembles the corresponding function of the armies of the capitalist state, but differs fundamentally from it in essence. The army of the exploiter state is used to suppress actions by the working people. The army of the socialist state suppresses insurrections of the exploiters, of the 'rebellious slave-owners' to use Lenin's words, and defends the revolutionary gains of the people.

The way in which this function is discharged depends on the conditions under which the socialist revolution is carried out; it may take the form of a war against the overthrown classes and foreign interventionists, or else of measures to prevent the outbreak of a civil war by foiling counter-revolutionary plots and rebellions, and by defeating armed counter-revolutionary gangs. . . .

In the course of their development the Armed Forces of the USSR have passed through two main stages. The first stage, during which they were an instrument of the socialist state, of the proletarian dictatorship, ends with the complete and final triumph of socialism in the country. During the present, second stage, the Armed Forces are an instrument of the socialist state of the whole people. These stages correspond to the character of the socio-economic and political relations dominant during these periods in the history of the Soviet people. At the same time they reflect the radical changes in the relation of forces in the world in favour of peace, democracy and socialism. . . .

Karl Marx and Frederick Engels advanced the idea of creating a proletarian military organisation of a new type. On the basis of an analysis and generalisation of the experience of the 1848–1849 revolution, and especially of the Paris Commune, they drew the conclusion that the first commandment of any victorious revolution is to smash the old army, to disband it, and to create a new one in its place. . . .

Before the October Revolution and immediately after its triumph, the Communist Party and the Soviet Government did not intend to create a regular army, but were guided by the Marxist proposition of replacing the regular army by a socialist militia. The armed intervention of international imperialism and the vast scope assumed by the Civil War made it necessary to revise this proposition. It was Lenin's great merit that he was the first Marxist courageously to advance and to lay a theoretical foundation for the idea that the Soviet state needed a regular army. . . .

At the Eighth Party Congress Lenin and his followers decisively rebuffed the 'army opposition', which was against strict discipline and centralised command of the army, insisted on a continuation of the partisan tactics inherited from the past, and thus obstructed the setting up of a regular army. The views of the 'army oppositon' were rejected and branded wrong and harmful. The Congress adopted Lenin's proposal to set up a regular Red Army. At the same time the Congress pointed out that it would be possible to make the transition to a socialist militia, when this would be warranted by the international situation.

A regular army is superior to the militia system. The troops of a regular army are much better trained, disciplined and organised.

The formations and units of the regular army are raised and stationed irrespective of the place of domicile and work of the draftees. Citizens called to the colours are freed from all other kinds of work for a long time, and military service becomes their main occupation. This makes it possible to organise their systematic training. The nucleus of the regular army is the cadre commanding echelon which is made up of professional soldiers. . . .

In the first years of the development of the Red Army, when a large number of ex-officers of the old tsarist army were among the commanders, and also in the headquarters while the Red commanders did not possess sufficient military-theoretical knowledge and experience in political work, a form of command had to be found that would serve the interests of the proletarian dictatorship and would at the same time suit the specific features of the military organisation. Dual command, under which a unit was headed by two persons—the commander and the commissar—was such a form.

During the Civil War and the foreign armed intervention the commissars played an exclusively important role in the formation and consolidation of the Red Army. They introduced organisation and iron proletarian discipline into the ranks, inspired them to heroism in action, consolidated them round the Bolshevik Party. In addition to carrying on Party-political work, the commissars supervised all the specific army activities—drill, administrative and logistic work, combat training, etc.

When alien and unworthy commanders had been weeded out and the political and military-theoretical level of commanders hailing from the working people had risen, it became unnecessary for two persons to deal simultaneously and in parallel with command, administrative and logistic questions. The increase in the share of Party members among the commanders, and the intense political education of the commanders created conditions for the merging of the two lines of command—the military and the political. Therefore, in keeping with the decisions of the Party CC, preparations were made for the introduction of one-man command throughout the army as early as 1924, and it was implemented in 1928....

Military discipline is an inalienable part of any army. Discipline in the Soviet Army differs radically from the discipline in the armies of exploiter states. Relations of co-operation and fraternal mutual assistance between the working people, and the social and political unity of the people, are the social basis of Soviet military discipline; communist consciousness, the understanding and conscious fulfilment by the servicemen of their military duty are its ideological basis.

Counterposing Soviet military discipline to the brutal and unthinking discipline in bourgeois armies, Lenin said: 'An army needs the strictest discipline. . . . The Red Army established unprecedentedly firm discipline—not by means of the lash, but based on the intelligence, loyalty and devotion of the workers and peasants themselves.

The numerical strength was determined in different epochs by the population figure, the development of material production, the social system and the financial possibilities of the state.

In the epoch of early feudalism the armies formed by knights were small (only from 800 to 1,000 knights took part in battles then considered big). The feudal decentralisation, the limited aims of wars, and the high cost of weapons prevented a growth in the numerical strength of the troops. During the period of absolute monarchies the armies generally did not exceed several tens of thousands of men because the state could not afford to support bigger armies.

The small strength of armies was also due to the difficulty of troop control in the absence of technical means of communication. Besides, the specifics of linear tactics, and the long drilling that was necessary to train the troops for combat, made it difficult to have large numbers of trained reserves.

Following the French bourgeois revolution, the armies grew much bigger, since recruiting was effected on the basis of conscription. Also, the more complicated equipment required preliminary training and the amassing of human reserves ready for action in case of war.

The armed forces of the belligerents reached great numerical strength during the Second World War. In modern conditions, when nuclear weapons and other means of destruction may be used, it is still necessary to have big regular armies. This is dictated by the character of modern war: the decisiveness of its aims, the unprecedentedly large territories involved, the complex and numerous equipment and weapons used, the high percentage of losses, the importance of defending the entire territory of the country in conditions when aerial means of destruction and air-borne landing forces will be used, the greater role of communications, their greater length and the necessity to defend them.

IV. THE TACTICS OF REVOLUTION

The enthusiasm of Marx and Engels during the 1840s for an audacious policy of proletarian insurrection against the bourgeois order gave way in subsequent years to the view that capitalism would be destroyed by its inner contradictions. What helped to bring about this change was the discovery by the French General Cavaignac in June 1848 of a successful method of dealing with the hitherto invulnerable barricades erected by the working men of Paris. From that time until the beginning of the new century, the Marxists, following Engels, saw the ballot, exercised by workers hard-pressed by capitalist exploitation, as the method by means of which a Socialist state would triumph. (See Section IVA, 1, 2, and Introduction.)

After the spontaneous adoption of a barricades strategy by the Russian working men in 1905, one which achieved a certain success, many Marxists reverted to the position of the 1840s, again seeing the usefulness of the 'art of insurrection', if properly guided by the Social-Democratic Party. Lenin (see Section IVA, 3) was among this number, as was also the more moderate intellectual leader of German Marxism, Karl Kautsky, the editor of the principal Marxist theoretical journal, *Die Neue Zeit*, and widely regarded as the heir to Engels's authority within the movement. Still, it was necessary to guard against the '"hooligan" perversion' of such spontaneous warfare, Lenin insisted, which would lead to a self-destructive anarchy.

Another issue which troubled Marx, Engels, and their followers was that of the usefulness of irregular warfare, modelled on the 'guerrilla' (little war) strategy adopted by bands of Spanish and Russian partisans against the invasions mounted by Napoleon's armies. In an 1854 article on the Spanish experience, the socialist theorists outlined a succession of strategies employed by the guerrillas according to the circumstances that prevailed in the various phases of the struggle (Section IVB, 1a)—constructing what might be called a sociology of guerrilla warfare.

In the light of the experience of the Opium War, which Britain waged against China between 1839 and 1842, the Anglo-Persian War of 1856 to 1858, and the renewal of hostilities between England and China as a result of the Arrow incident in 1856, Marx and Engels came to certain conclusions about how Asians might counter intrusions by western armies. In the Opium War, the Chinese armies organized under oriental principles had proved no match for a westernized Anglo-Indian army. In Persia, an Asian army had been unsuccessful in its efforts to organize itself to fight on the Western plan. However, in China, in 1856 and 1857, a new system of tactics was employed by the Chinese populace: mobs pillaged foreign warehouses and terrorized European residents. In Asia, Marx and Engels suggested, guerrilla tactics might be the best method to employ against Western armies. (Section IVB, 1b.) In 1857 and 1858, sections of the Anglo-Indian army, which had hitherto proved so effective in Persia and India, rose in mutiny against their officers. Native princes and their forces joined in this insurrection against the British. The still-loyal forces of the Anglo-Indian army moved decisively and at times brutally, against the rebel Sepoys. Marx and Engels wrote many articles discussing the events of the mutiny. In several, they predicted, as it happens incorrectly, that after the defeat of their main forces, the Indians would mount a wounding guerrilla campaign against the British regulars. (Section IVB, 1c.) In 1860, again writing in the *Tribune*, Marx and Engels described the guerrilla warfare actually waged against the Spaniards in their Moroccan colony. In these articles, however, the successes of the guerrillas were explained away by the socialist theorists on the grounds of ineffectiveness of the Spanish army and its generals. A guerrilla force, Marx and Engels suggested, was no match for a properly-led western army. (Section IVB, 1d.) Finally, in 1870, in the course of the war between France and Prussia, Engels more hopefully surveyed the successes of the French guerrillas against the invading Prussian armies. (Section IVB, 1e.) All in all, Marx and

Engels, while seeing the strength of a guerrilla strategy, both in Asia and in Europe, were far from certain that it could effectively counter a well-led, efficiently organized modern army.

After the inconclusive Revolution of 1905 in Russia—which erupted after the frustrating defeats which the Tsar's forces encountered in Russia's war with Japan, then in progress—Lenin gave a more thoroughgoing attention to the usefulness of guerrilla war. At this time (Section IVB, 2), Lenin took issue with the Marxist 'systematizers' who 'in the seclusion of their studies' had described irregular warfare as opposed to Marxist tenets. In order to decide on the usefulness of a set of tactics, a Marxist must make 'a detailed examination of the concrete situation of the given movement at the given stage of development'. All in all, in 1906, Lenin argued not so much for guerrilla strategy, which he never fully trusted since irregular forces might too readily get out of control, but in opposition to a doctrinaire dismissal of such a strategy. In the course of the Russian Civil War of 1918 and 1922, fought between the Bolshevik forces and the White Armies seeking to overthrow the Soviet regime, Lenin supported Trotsky's military programme against the attacks of a new generation of Marxist systematizers who now saw a guerrilla strategy as the only properly Marxist strategy. The systematizers were particularly unhappy with the traditional strategy of 'positionalism' to which they opposed one of 'manœuvre'. Trotsky defended a pragmatic policy, the use of whatever tactics seemed appropriate to the prevailing conditions, and ridiculed those who called for a 'proletarian military doctrine'. (Section IVB, 3.)

The same issue emerged in the early years of the Chinese Revolution, when the Li Li-san faction of the Chinese Communist party insisted that a Marxist must adopt the strategy of mounting proletarian uprisings in the cities. In line with nineteenth-century Marxism, Li and his associates denounced guerrilla tactics, which they saw as anarchist, in favour of an orderly positionalism. Mao Tse-tung, who was to become the communist leader in the mid-thirties, defended a pragmatic policy, which in the prevailing circumstances meant a policy of manœuvre and guerrilla warfare in the countryside, and above all avoiding a decisive engagement which might destroy the Red Army. (Section IVB, 4a,b,c.)

Leon Trotsky, in his battle with the 'systematizers' of 1918-22, had warned that generalizing a guerrilla strategy might undermine revolutions in Europe where a more traditional strategy would probably prove more effective. (Section IVC, 1.) After the victory of the Red Armies in China, what had first been presented by Mao as a pragmatic military doctrine became a new orthodoxy, and Mao and his followers were prepared to recommend its universal adoption by Marxists. Such a generalization of guerrilla strategy, which Trotsky feared, was made by Mao's chosen successor, Lin Piao, who based his strategy of the coming communist triumph over capitalism upon the tactics pursued by Mao in the 1930s and 1940s. (Section IVC, 2.)

Lin Piao (1908-71), the son of a Hupeh factory owner, was a veteran of the 'Long March' of 1934-5, and served successfully as a commander against both the forces of Chiang's Nationalists and the Japanese. After many years of activity in both military and political positions, he became both a Marshal of the Chinese People's Republic and a member of the Communist Politburo in 1955. In mid-1965, clearly at Mao's behest, Lin restored the army to the 'internal democracy' of the guerrilla days by abolishing all military ranks. In the following year, when the Cultural Revolution was launched, Lin assumed charge of the Red Guards, and was rewarded by being named Mao's heir-designate. Lin was killed in an aeroplane crash in 1971, under suspicious circumstances. It was later suggested that he had been assassinated just as he was on the point of carrying out a pro-Soviet coup in China.

The Frenchman Régis Debray (1942-), a student of the Marxist philosopher Louis Althusser, went to teach in Cuba after the successful revolution of 1959. Debray's tracts on the tactics of a guerrilla war were based upon the strategy actually pursued by the Cuban military leader, Fidel Castro, and his chief associate, the Argentinian-born Che Guevara (1928-67) against the Batista regime. Debray was to set off with Guevara to mount a revolution in the Bolivian Andes in the mid-1960s. Guevara was killed by government troops in 1967, and Debray captured and imprisoned. After his release, he returned to France, and a literary career.

Debray has formulated a military model of Marxism-Leninism, in opposition to what he described as the 'medieval metaphysic' of classical Marxist doctrine. Like Lin, he favored a guerrilla strategy, though somewhat different from that pursued by Mao. What seemed most startling was his expectation that the guerrilla military leaders, tested in battle and proletarianized by years of guerrilla warfare, would become the political leaders of the communist state after the victory of the revolution. Rather than denouncing this realization of the Cromwellian and Napoleonic nightmare of Marx, Engels, and Lenin, Debray cheered. (Section IVC, 3.) In the 1970s, these views were similarly welcomed, along with Cuban soldiers, by the Marxist leaders of Angola and Ethiopia. (See Introduction.)

IVA. 'To the Barricades!'

*1. Marx and Engels, 'Insurrection as an Art'**

Now, insurrection is an art quite as much as war or any other, and subject to certain rules of proceeding, which, when neglected, will produce the ruin of the party neglecting them. Those rules, logical deductions from the nature of the parties and the circumstances one has to deal with in such a case, are so plain and simple that the short experience of 1848 had made the Germans pretty well acquainted with them. Firstly, never play with insurrection unless you are fully prepared to face the consequences of your play. Insurrection is a calculus with very indefinite magnitudes, the value of which may change every day; the forces opposed to you have all the advantage of organization, discipline, and habitual authority; unless you bring strong odds against them you are defeated and ruined. Secondly, the insurrectionary career once entered upon, act with the greatest determination, and on the offensive. The defensive is the death of every armed rising; it is lost before it measures itself with its enemies. Surprise your antagonists while their forces are scattering, prepare new successes, however small, but daily; keep up the moral ascendency which

* Excerpts from K. Marx and F. Engels, article in *New York Daily Tribune*, Sept. 18 1852. [Republished in F. Engels, *Germany: Revolution and Counter-Revolution* (New York: International Publishers, 1933), p. 100.]

the first successful rising has given to you; rally those vacillating elements to your side which always follow the strongest impulse, and which always look out for the safer side; force your enemies to a retreat before they can collect their strength against you; in the words of Danton, the greatest master of revolutionary policy yet known, *de l'audace, de l'audace, encore de l'audace!*

*IVA, 2. Engels, 'The Tactics of the Barricade'**

With successful utilization of universal suffrage, an entirely new mode of proletarian struggle came into force, and this quickly developed further. It was found that the state institutions, in which the rule of the bourgeoisie is organized, offer still further opportunities for the working class to fight these very state institutions. They took part in elections to individual diets, to municipal councils and to industrial courts; they contested every post against the bourgeoisie in the occupation of which a sufficient part of the proletariat had its say. And so it happened that the bourgeoisie and the government came to be much more afraid of the legal than of the illegal action of the workers' party, of the results of elections than of those of rebellion.

For here, too, the conditions of the struggle had essentially changed. Rebellion in the old style, the street fight with barricades, which up to 1848 gave everywhere the final decision, was to a considerable extent obsolete.

Let us have no illusions about it: a real victory of an insurrection over the military in street fighting, a victory as between two armies, is one of the rarest exceptions. But the insurgents, also, counted on it just as rarely. For them it was solely a question of making the troops yield to moral influences, which, in a fight between the armies of two warring countries, do not come into play at all, or do so to a much less degree. If they succeed in this, then the troops fail to act, or the commanding officers lose their heads, and the insurrection wins. If they do not succeed in this, then, even where the military are in the minority, the superiority of better equipment and training, of unified leadership, of the planned employment of

* F. Engels, 'Introduction' (1895) to K. Marx, *The Class Struggles in France, 1848-50* (New York: International Publishers, 1964), pp. 21-5.

the military forces and of discipline makes itself felt. The most that the insurrection can achieve in actual tactical practice is the correct construction and defense of a single barricade. Mutual support; the disposition and employment of reserves; in short, the co-operation and harmonious working of the individual detachments, indispensable even for the defense of one quarter of the town, not to speak of the whole of a large town, are at best defective, and mostly not attainable at all; concentration of the military forces at a decisive point is, of course, impossible. Hence the passive defense is the prevailing form of fight: the attack will rise here and there, but only by way of exception, to occasional advances and flank assaults; as a rule, however, it will be limited to occupation of the positions abandoned by the retreating troops. In addition, the military have, on their side, the disposal of artillery and fully equipped corps of skilled engineers, resources of war which, in nearly every case, the insurgents entirely lack. No wonder, then, that even the barricade struggles conducted with the greatest heroism—Paris, June 1848; Vienna, October 1848; Dresden, May 1849—ended with the defeat of the insurrection, so soon as the leaders of the attack, unhampered by political considerations, acted from the purely military standpoint, and their soldiers remained reliable.

The numerous successes of the insurgents up to 1848 were due to a great variety of causes. In Paris in July 1830 and February 1848, as in most of the Spanish street fights, there stood between the insurgents and the military a civic militia, which either directly took the side of the insurrection, or else by its lukewarm, indecisive attitude caused the troops likewise to vacillate, and supplied the insurrection with arms into the bargain. Where this citizens' guard opposed the insurrection from the outset, as in June 1848 in Paris, the insurrection was vanquished. In Berlin in 1848, the people were victorious partly through a considerable accession of new fighting forces during the night and the morning of the 19th, partly as a result of the exhaustion and bad victualing of the troops, and, finally, partly as a result of the paralyzed command. But in all cases the fight was won because the troops failed to obey, because the officers had lost their power of decision or because their hands were tied.

Even in the classic time of street fighting, therefore, the barricade produced more of a moral than a material effect. It was a means of shaking the steadfastness of the military. If it held out until this was attained, then victory was won; if not, there was defeat. This is the main point, which must be kept in view, likewise when the chances of contingent future street fights are examined.

The chances, however, were in 1849 already pretty poor. Everywhere the bourgeoisie had thrown in its lot with the governments, 'culture and property' had hailed and feasted the military moving against the insurrections. The spell of the barricade was broken; the soldier no longer saw behind it 'the people,' but rebels, agitators, plunderers, levelers, the scum of society; the officer had in the course of time become versed in the tactical forms of street fighting, he no longer marched straight ahead and without cover against the improvised breastwork, but went round it through gardens, yards and houses. And this was now successful, with a little skill, in nine cases out of ten.

But since then there have been very many more changes, and all in favor of the military. If the big towns have become considerably bigger, the armies have become bigger still. Paris and Berlin have, since 1848, grown less than fourfold, but their garrisons have grown more than that. By means of the railways, the garrisons can, in 24 hours, be more than doubled, and in 48 hours they can be increased to huge armies. The arming of this enormously increased number of troops has become incomparably more effective. In 1848 the smoothbore percussion muzzle-loader, today the small-caliber magazine breech-loading rifle, which shoots four times as far, ten times as accurately and ten times as fast as the former. At that time the relatively ineffective round-shot and grape-shot of the artillery; today the percussion shells, of which one is sufficient to demolish the best barricade. At that time the pickaxe of the sapper for breaking through walls; today the dynamite cartridge.

On the other hand, all the conditions on the insurgents' side have grown worse. An insurrection with which all sections of the people sympathize will hardly recur; in the class struggle all the middle sections will never group themselves round the proletariat so exclusively that the reactionary parties gathered round the bourgeoisie well-nigh disappear. The 'people,' therefore, will always appear divided, and with this a powerful lever, so extraordinarily effective in 1848, is lacking. Even if more soldiers who have seen service were to come over to the insurrectionists, the arming of them becomes so much the more difficult. The hunting and luxury guns of the gun shops—even if not previously made unusable by removal of part of the lock by the police—are far from being a match for the magazine rifle of the soldier, even in close fighting. Up to 1848 it was possible to make the necessary ammunition oneself out of powder and lead; today the cartridges differ for each rifle, and are everywhere alike only in one point, that they are a special product of big industry, and therefore not to be prepared *ex tempore* [on the spur of the moment], with the result that most rifles are useless as long as one does not possess the ammunition specially suited to them. And, finally, since 1848 the newly built quarters of the big towns have been laid out in long, straight, broad streets, as though made to give full effect to the new cannons and rifles. The revolutionary would have to be mad, who himself chose the working-class districts in the North and East of Berlin for a barricade fight. Does that mean that in the future the street fight will play no further role? Certainly not. It only means that the conditions since 1848 have become far more unfavorable for civil fights, far more favorable for the military. A future street fight can therefore only be victorious when this unfavorable situation is compensated by other factors. Accordingly, it will occur more seldom in the beginning of a great revolution than in its further progress, and will have to be undertaken with greater forces. These, however, may then well prefer, as in the whole Great French Revolution or on September 4 and October 31, 1870, in Paris, the open attack to the passive barricade tactics.

Does the reader now understand why the ruling classes decidedly want to bring us to where the guns shoot and the sabers slash? Why they accuse us today of cowardice, because we do not betake ourselves without more ado into the street, where we are certain of defeat in advance? Why they so earnestly implore us to play for once the part of cannon fodder?

The gentlemen pour out their prayers and their challenges

for nothing, for nothing at all. We are not so stupid. They might just as well demand from their enemy in the next war that he should take up his position in the line formation of old Fritz [Frederick the Great of Prussia], or in the columns of whole divisions *à la* Wagram and Waterloo, and with the flintlock in his hands at that. If the conditions have changed in the case of war between nations, this is no less true in the case of class struggle. The time of surprise attacks, of revolutions carried through by small conscious minorities at the head of the unconscious masses, is past. Where it is a question of a complete transformation of the social organization, the masses themselves must be also in it, must themselves already have grasped what is at stake, what they are going in for with body and soul. The history of the last 50 years has taught us that. But in order that the masses may understand what is to be done, long, persistent work is required, and it is just this work which we are now pursuing, and with a success that drives the enemy to despair.

*IVA, 3. Lenin, 'The Lessons of the Moscow Uprising of 1905'**

The December action in Moscow vividly demonstrated that the general strike, as an independent and predominant form of struggle, is out of date, that the movement is breaking out of these narrow bounds with elemental and irresistible force and giving rise to the highest form of struggle—an uprising.

In calling the strike, all the revolutionary parties, all the Moscow unions recognized and even intuitively felt that it must inevitably grow into an uprising. On December 6 the Soviet of Workers' Deputies resolved to 'strive to transform the strike into an armed uprising.' As a matter of fact, however, none of the organizations were prepared for this. Even the Joint Council of Volunteer Fighting Squads spoke (*on December 9!*) of an uprising as of something remote, and it is quite evident that it had no hand in or control of the street fighting that took place. The organizations *failed to keep pace* with the growth and range of the movement.

The strike was growing into an uprising, primarily as a result

* Excerpts from V. I. Lenin, 'The Lessons of the Moscow Uprising of 1905' (1906), in *Selected Works* (New York: International Publishers, 1967), I: 577–83. [First published in *Proletary*, Aug. 29 1906.]

of the pressure of the objective conditions created after October. A general strike could no longer take the government unawares: it had already organized the forces of counter-revolution, and they were ready for military action. The whole course of the Russian revolution after October, and the sequence of events in Moscow in the December days, strikingly confirmed one of Marx's profound propositions: revolution progresses by giving rise to a strong and united counter-revolution, i.e., it compels the enemy to resort to more and more extreme measures of defense and in this way devises ever more powerful means of attack.

December 7 and 8: a peaceful strike, peaceful mass demonstrations. Evening of the 8th: the siege of the Aquarium. The morning of the 9th: the crowd in Strastnaya Square is attacked by the dragoons. Evening: the Fiedler building is raided. Temper rises. The unorganized street crowds, quite spontaneously and hesitatingly, set up the first barricades.

The 10th: artillery fire is opened on the barricades and the crowds in the streets. Barricades are set up more deliberately, and no longer in isolated cases, but on a really mass scale. The whole population is in the streets: all the main centers of the city are covered by a network of barricades. For several days the volunteer fighting units wage a stubborn guerrilla battle against the troops, which exhausts the troops and compels Dubasov [Military Governor-General of Moscow] to beg for reinforcements. Only on December 15 did the superiority of the government forces become complete, and on December 17 the Semyonovsky Regiment crushed Presnya District, the last stronghold of the uprising.

From a strike and demonstrations to isolated barricades. From isolated barricades to the mass erection of barricades and street fighting against the troops. Over the heads of the organizations, the mass proletarian struggle developed from a strike to an uprising. This is the greatest historic gain the Russian revolution achieved in December 1905; and like all preceding gains it was purchased at the price of enormous sacrifices. The movement was raised from a general political strike to a higher stage. It compelled the reaction to go *to the limit* in its resistance, and so brought vastly nearer the moment when the revolution will also go to the limit in applying the means of attack. The reaction *cannot* go further than the shelling of barricades, buildings and crowds. But the revolution can go very much further than the Moscow volunteer fighting units; it can go very, very much further in breadth and depth. And the revolution has advanced far since December. The base of the revolutionary crisis has become immeasurably broader—the blade must now be sharpened to a keener edge.

The proletariat sensed sooner than its leaders the change in the objective conditions of the struggle and the need for a transition from the strike to an uprising. As is always the case, practice marched ahead of theory. A peaceful strike and demonstrations immediately ceased to satisfy the workers; they asked: What is to be done next? And they demanded more resolute action. The instructions to set up barricades reached the districts exceedingly late, when barricades were already being erected in the center of the city. The workers set to work in large numbers, but *even this did not satisfy them*; they wanted to know: what is to be done next?—they demanded active measures. In December, we, the leaders of the Social-Democratic proletariat, were like a commander-in-chief who has deployed his troops in such an absurd way that most of them took no active part in the battle. The masses of the workers demanded, but failed to receive, instructions for resolute mass action.

Thus, nothing could be more short-sighted than Plekhanov's view, seized upon by all the opportunists, that the strike was untimely and should not have been started, and that 'they should not have taken to arms.' On the contrary, we should have taken to arms more resolutely, energetically and aggressively; we should have explained to the masses that it was impossible to confine things to a peaceful strike and that a fearless and relentless armed fight was necessary. And now we must at last openly and publicly admit that political strikes are inadequate; we must carry on the widest agitation among the masses in favor of an armed uprising and make no attempt to obscure this question by talk about 'preliminary stages,' or to befog it in any way. We would be deceiving both ourselves and the people if we concealed from the masses the necessity of a desperate, bloody war of extermination, as the immediate task of the coming revolutionary action.

Such is the first lesson of the December events. Another lesson concerns the character of the uprising, the methods by which it is conducted, and the conditions which lead to the troops coming over to the side of the people. An extremely biased view on this latter point prevails in the right wing of our party. It is alleged that there is no possibility of fighting modern troops; the troops must become revolutionary. Of course, unless the revolution assumes a mass character and affects the troops, there can be no question of serious struggle. That we must work among the troops goes without saying. But we must not imagine that they will come over to our side at one stroke, as a result of persuasion or their own convictions. The Moscow uprising clearly demonstrated how stereotyped and lifeless this view is. As a matter of fact, the wavering of the troops, which is inevitable in every truly popular movement, leads to a real *fight for the troops* whenever the revolutionary struggle becomes acute. The Moscow uprising was precisely an example of the desperate, frantic struggle for the troops that takes place between the reaction and the revolution. Dubasov himself declared that of the 15,000 men of the Moscow garrison, only 5,000 were reliable. The government restrained the waverers by the most diverse and desperate measures: they appealed to them, flattered them, bribed them, presented them with watches, money, etc.: they doped them with vodka, they lied to them, threatened them, confined them to barracks and disarmed them, and those who were suspected of being least reliable were removed by treachery and violence. And we must have the courage to confess, openly and unreservedly, that in this respect we lagged behind the government. We failed to utilize the forces at our disposal for such an active, bold, resourceful and aggressive fight for the wavering troops as that which the government waged and won. We have carried on work in the army and we will redouble our efforts in the future ideologically to 'win over' the troops. But we shall prove to be miserable pedants if we forget that at a time of uprising there must also be a physical struggle for the troops.

In the December days, the Moscow proletariat taught us magnificent lessons in ideologically 'winning over' the troops, as, for example, on December 8 in Strastnaya Square, when the crowd surrounded the Cossacks, mingled and fraternized with them, and persuaded them to turn back. Or on December 10, in Presnya District, when two working girls, carrying a red flag in a crowd of 10,000 people, rushed out to meet the Cossacks crying: 'Kill us! We shall not surrender the flag alive!' And the Cossacks were disconcerted and galloped away, amidst the shouts from the crowd: 'Hurrah for the Cossacks!' These examples of courage and heroism should be impressed forever on the mind of the proletariat.

But here are examples of how we lagged behind Dubasov. On December 9, soldiers were marching down Bolshaya Serpukhovskaya Street singing the *Marseillaise*, on their way to join the insurgents. The workers sent delegates to meet them. Malakhov [Chief of Staff of the Moscow Military Area] himself galloped at breakneck speed toward them. The workers were too late, Malakhov reached them first. He delivered a passionate speech, caused the soldiers to waver, surrounded them with dragoons, marched them off to barracks and locked them in. Malakhov reached the soldiers in time and we did not, although within two days 150,000 people had risen at our call, and these could and should have organized the patrolling of the streets. Malakhov surrounded the soldiers with dragoons, whereas we failed to surround the Malakhovs with bomb-throwers. We could and should have done this; and long ago the Social-Democratic press (the old *Iskra*) pointed out that ruthless extermination of civil and military chiefs was our duty during an uprising. What took place in Bolshaya Serpukhovskaya Street was apparently repeated in its main features in front of the Nesvizhskiye Barracks and the Krutitskiye Barracks, and also when the workers attempted to 'withdraw' the Ekaterinoslav Regiment, and when delegates were sent to the sappers in Alexandrov, and when the Rostov artillery on its way to Moscow was turned back, and when the sappers were disarmed in Kolomna, and so on. During the uprising we proved unequal to our task in the fight for the wavering troops.

The December events confirmed another of Marx's profound propositions, which the opportunists have forgotten, namely, that insurrection is an art and that the principal rule of this art is the waging of a desperately bold and irrevocably determined *offensive*. We have not sufficiently assimilated this truth. We ourselves have not sufficiently learned, nor have we taught the masses, this art, this rule to attack at all costs. We must make up for this omission with all our energy. It is not enough to take sides on the question of political slogans; it is also necessary to take sides on the question of an armed uprising. Those who are opposed to it, those who do not prepare for it, must be ruthlessly dismissed from the ranks of the supporters of the revolution, sent packing to its enemies, to the traitors or cowards; for the day is approaching when the force of events and the conditions of the struggle will compel us to distinguish between enemies and friends according to this principle. It is not passivity that we should preach, not mere 'waiting' until the troops 'come over.' No! We must proclaim from the housetops the need for a bold offensive and armed attack, the necessity at such times of exterminating the persons in command of the enemy, and of a most energetic fight for the wavering troops.

The third great lesson taught by Moscow concerns the tactics and organization of the forces for an uprising. Military tactics depend on the level of military technique. This plain truth Engels demonstrated and brought home to all Marxists. Military technique today is not what it was in the middle of the 19th century. It would be folly to contend against artillery in crowds and defend barricades with revolvers. Kautsky was right when he wrote that it is high time now, after Moscow, to review Engels' conclusions, and that Moscow had inaugurated '*new barricade tactics.*' These tactics are the tactics of guerrilla warfare. The organization required for such tactics is that of mobile and exceedingly small units, units of ten, three or even two persons. We often meet Social-Democrats now who scoff whenever units of five or three are mentioned. But scoffing is only a cheap way of ignoring the *new* question of tactics and organization raised by street fighting under the conditions imposed by modern military technique. Study carefully the story of the Moscow uprising, gentlemen, and you will understand what connection exists between 'units of five' and the question of 'new barricade tactics.'

Moscow advanced these tactics, but failed to develop them far enough, to apply them to any considerable extent, to a really mass extent. There were too few volunteer fighting squads, the slogan of bold attack was not issued to the masses of the workers and they did not apply it; the guerrilla detachments were too uniform in character, their arms and methods were inadequate, their ability to lead the crowd was almost undeveloped. We must make up for all this and we shall do so by learning from the experience of Moscow, by spreading this experience among the masses and by stimulating their creative efforts to develop it still further. And the guerrilla warfare and mass terror that have been taking place throughout Russia practically without a break since December, will undoubtedly help the masses to learn the correct tactics of an uprising. Social-Democracy must recognize this mass terror and incorporate it into its tactics, organizing and controlling it of course, subordinating it to the interests and conditions of the working-class movement and the general revolutionary struggle, while eliminating and ruthlessly lopping off the 'hooligan' perversion of this guerrilla warfare which was so splendidly and ruthlessly dealt with by our Moscow comrades during the uprising and by the Letts during the days of the famous Lettish republics.

There have been new advances in military technique in the very recent period. The Japanese War produced the hand grenade. The small-arms factories have placed automatic rifles on the market. Both these weapons are already being successfully used in the Russian revolution, but to a degree that is far from adequate. We can and must take advantage of improvements in technique, teach the workers' detachments to make bombs in large quantities, help them and our fighting squads to obtain supplies of explosives, fuses and automatic rifles. If the mass of workers takes part in uprisings in the towns, if mass attacks are launched on the enemy, if a determined and skillful fight is waged for the troops who, after the Duma, after Sveaborg and Kronstadt, are wavering more than ever—and if we ensure participation of the rural areas in the general struggle—victory will be ours in the next all-Russian armed uprising.

Let us, then, develop our work more extensively and set our tasks more boldly, while mastering the lessons of the great days of the Russian revolution. The basis of our work is a correct estimate of class interests and of the requirements of the nation's development at the present juncture. We are rallying, and shall continue to rally, an increasing section of the proletariat, the peasantry and the army under the slogan of overthrowing the tsarist regime and convening a constituent assembly by a revolutionary government. As hitherto, the basis and chief content of our work is to develop the political understanding of the masses. But let us not forget that, in addition to this general, constant and fundamental task, times like the present in Russia impose other, particular and special tasks. Let us not become pedants and philistines, let us not evade these special tasks of the moment, these special tasks of the given forms of struggle, by meaningless references to our permanent duties, which remain unchanged at all times and in all circumstances.

Let us remember that a great mass struggle is approaching. It will be an armed uprising. It must, as far as possible, be simultaneous. The masses must know that they are entering upon an armed, bloody and desperate struggle. Contempt for death must become widespread among them and will ensure victory. The onslaught on the enemy must be pressed with the greatest vigor; attack, not defense, must be the slogan of the masses; the ruthless extermination of the enemy will be their task; the organization of the struggle will become mobile and flexible; the wavering elements among the troops will be drawn into active participation. And in this momentous struggle, the party of the class-conscious proletariat must discharge its duty to the full.

IVB. Guerrilla Warfare vs. Regular Warfare

1. Marx and Engels on Guerrilla War

*a. 'Guerrilla War in Spain'** There are three periods to be distinguished in the history of the guerrilla warfare. In the first period the population of whole provinces took up arms and made partisan warfare, as in Galicia and Asturias. In the second period, guerrilla bands formed of the wrecks of the Spanish armies, of Spanish deserters from the French armies,

* Excerpts from K. Marx and F. Engels, article in *New York Daily Tribune*, Oct. 30 1854. [Republished in K. Marx and F. Engels, *Revolution in Spain* (International Publishers, 1939), pp. 51-5.]

of smugglers, etc., carried on the war as their own cause, independently of all foreign influence and agreeable to their immediate interest. Fortunate events and circumstances frequently brought whole districts under their colors. As long as the guerrillas were thus constituted, they made no formidable appearance as a body, but were nevertheless extremely dangerous to the French. They formed the basis of an actual armament of the people. As soon as an opportunity for a capture offered itself, or a combined enterprise was meditated, the most active and daring among the people came out and joined the guerrillas. They rushed with the utmost rapidity upon their booty, or placed themselves in order of battle, according to the object of their undertaking. It was not uncommon to see them standing out a whole day in sight of a vigilant enemy, in order to intercept a courier or to capture supplies. It was in this way that the younger Mina captured the Viceroy of Navarra, appointed by Joseph Bonaparte, and that Julian made a prisoner of the Commandante of Ciudad Rodrigo. As soon as the enterprise was completed, everybody went his own way, and armed men were soon scattering in all directions; but the associated peasants quietly returned to their common occupation without 'as much as their absence having been noticed.' Thus the communication on all the roads was closed. Thousands of enemies were on the spot, though not one could be discovered. No courier could be dispatched without being taken; no supplies could set out without being intercepted; in short, no movement could be effected without being observed by a hundred eyes. At the same time, there existed no means of striking at the root of a combination of this kind. The French were obliged to be constantly armed against an enemy who, continually flying, always reappeared, and was everywhere without being actually seen, the mountains serving as so many curtains. 'It was,' says the Abbéde Pradt, 'neither battles nor engagements which exhausted the French forces, but the incessant molestations of an invisible enemy, who, if pursued, became lost among the people, out of which he reappeared immediately afterward with renewed strength. The lion in the fable tormented to death by a gnat gives a true picture of the French army.' In their third period, the guerrillas aped the regularity of the standing army, swelled their corps to the number of from 3,000 to 6,000 men, ceased to be the concern of whole districts, and fell into the hands of a few leaders, who made such use of them as best suited their own purposes. This change in the system of the guerrillas gave the French, in their contests with them, considerable advantage. Rendered incapable by their great numbers to conceal themselves, and to suddenly disappear without being forced into battle, as they had formerly done, the *guerrilleros* were now frequently overtaken, defeated, dispersed, and disabled for a length of time from offering any further molestation.

By comparing the three periods of guerrilla warfare with the political history of Spain, it is found that they represent the respective degrees into which the counter-revolutionary spirit of the government had succeeded in cooling the spirit of the people. Beginning with the rise of whole populations, the partisan war was next carried on by guerrilla bands, of which whole districts formed the reserve and terminated in *corps francs* (commandos) continually on the point of dwindling into *banditti*, or sinking down to the level of standing regiments.

Estrangement from the Supreme Government, relaxed discipline, continual disasters, constant formation, decomposition, and recomposition during six years of the *cadrez* must have necessarily stamped upon the body of the Spanish army the character of praetorianism, making them equally ready to become the tools or the scourges of their chiefs. The generals themselves had necessarily participated in, quarreled with, or conspired against the central government, and always thrown the weight of their sword into the political balance. . . .

On the other hand, the army and *guerrilleros*—which received during the war part of their chiefs, like Porlier, Lacy, Eroles and Villacampa, from the ranks of distinguished officers of the line, while the line in its turn afterward received guerrilla chiefs, like Mina, Empecinado, etc.—were the most revolutionized portion of Spanish society, recruited as they were from all ranks, including the whole of the fiery, aspiring and patriotic youth, inaccessible to the soporific influence of the central government; emancipated from the shackles of the ancient regime; part of them, like Riego, returning after some years' captivity in France. We are, then, not to be surprised at the influence exercised by the Spanish army in subsequent commotions; neither when taking the revolutionary initiative, nor when spoiling the revolution by praetorianism.

As to the guerrillas, it is evident that, having for some years figured upon the theater of sanguinary contests, taken to roving habits, freely indulged all the passions of hatred, revenge and love of plunder, they must, in times of peace, form a most dangerous mob, always ready at a nod in the name of any party or principle, to step forward for him who is able to give them good pay or to afford them a pretext for plundering excursions.

*IVB, 1b. Marx and Engels, 'On Western Military Technique in Asia'** The English have just concluded an Asiatic war, and are entering upon another. The resistance offered by the Persians, and that which the Chinese have so far opposed to British invasion, form a contrast worth our attention. In Persia, the European system of military organization has been engrafted upon Asiatic barbarity; in China, the rotting semi-civilization of the oldest State in the world meets the Europeans with its own resources. Persia has been signally defeated, while distracted, half-dissolved China has hit upon a system of resistance which, if followed up, will render impossible repetition of the triumphal marches of the first Anglo-Chinese war....

The fact is that the introduction of European military organization with barbaric nations is far from being completed when the new army has been subdivided, equipped and drilled after the European fashion. That is merely the first step toward it. Nor will the enactment of some European military code suffice; it will no more ensure European discipline than a European set of drill-regulations will produce, by itself, European tactics and strategy. The main point, and at the same time the main difficulty, is the creation of a body of officers and sergeants, educated on the modern European system, totally freed from the old national prejudices and reminiscences in military matters, and fit to inspire life into

* Excerpts from K. Marx and F. Engels, article in *New York Daily Tribune*, May 22 1857. [Republished in K. Marx and F. Engels, *On Colonialism* (Moscow, n.d.), pp. 123-7.]

the new formation. This requires a long time, and is sure to meet with the most obstinate opposition from Oriental ignorance, impatience, prejudice, and the vicissitudes of fortune and favour inherent to Eastern courts. A Sultan or Shah is but too apt to consider his army equal to anything as soon as the men can defile in parade, wheel, deploy and form column without getting into hopeless disorder. And as to military schools, their fruits are so slow in ripening that under the instabilities of Eastern governments they can scarcely ever be expected to show any. Even in Turkey, the supply of educated officers is but scanty, and the Turkish army could not have done at all, during the late war, without the great number of renegades and the European officers in its ranks.

The only arm which everywhere forms an exception is the artillery. Here the Orientals are so much at fault and so helpless that they have to leave the whole management to their European instructors. The consequence is that as in Turkey, so in Persia, the artillery was far ahead of the infantry and cavalry.

That under these circumstances the Anglo-Indian army, the oldest of all Eastern armies organized on the European system, the only one that is subject not to an Eastern, but an exclusively European government, and officered almost entirely by Europeans—that this army, supported by a strong reserve of British troops and a powerful navy, should easily disperse the Persian regulars, is but a matter of course. The reverse will do the Persians the more good the more signal it was. They will now see, as the Turks have seen before, that European dress and parade-drill is no talisman in itself, and maybe, twenty years hence, the Persians will turn out as respectable as the Turks did in their late victories.

The troops which conquered Bushire and Mohammerah will, it is understood, be at once sent to China. There they will find a different enemy. No attempts at European evolutions, but the irregular array of Asiatic masses, will oppose them there. Of these they no doubt will easily dispose; but what if the Chinese wage against them a national war, and if barbarism be unscrupulous enough to use the only weapons which it knows how to wield?

There is evidently a different spirit among the Chinese now

to what they showed in the war of 1840 to 1842. Then, the people were quiet; they left the Emperor's soldiers to fight the invaders, and submitted after a defeat with Eastern fatalism to the power of the enemy. But now, at least in the southern provinces, to which the contest has so far been confined, the mass of the people take an active, nay, a fanatical part in the struggle against the foreigners. They poison the bread of the European community at Hongkong by wholesale, and with the coolest premeditation. . . . They go with hidden arms on board trading steamers, and, when on the journey, massacre the crew and European passengers and seize the boat. They kidnap and kill every foreigner within their reach. The very coolies emigrating to foreign countries rise in mutiny, and as if by concert, on board every emigrant ship, and fight for its possession, and, rather than surrender, go down to the bottom with it, or perish in its flames. Even out of China, the Chinese colonists, the most submissive and meek of subjects hitherto, conspire and suddenly rise in nightly insurrection, as at Sarawak; or, as at Singapore, are held down by main force and vigilance only. The piratical policy of the British Government has caused this universal outbreak of all Chinese against all foreigners, and marked it as a war of extermination.

What is an army to do against a people resorting to such means of warfare? Where, how far, is it to penetrate into the enemy's country, how to maintain itself there? Civilization-mongers who throw hot shell on a defenceless city and add rape to murder, may call the system cowardly, barbarous, atrocious; but what matters it to the Chinese if it be only successful? Since the British treat them as barbarians, they cannot deny to them the full benefit of their barbarism. If their kidnappings, surprises, midnight massacres are what we call cowardly, the civilization-mongers should not forget that according to their own showing they could not stand against European means of destruction with their ordinary means of warfare.

*IVB, 1c. Marx and Engels, 'The Possibility of Guerrilla War in India'** May 25 1858—We are also informed that among the British officers the opinion is gaining ground that the guerrilla warfare which is sure to succeed the dispersion of the larger bodies of insurgents, will be far more harassing and destructive of life to the British than the present war with its battles and sieges. And, lastly, the Sikhs are beginning to talk in a way which bodes no good to the English. They feel that without their assistance the British would scarcely have been able to hold India, and that, had they joined the insurrection, Hindostan would certainly have been lost to England, at least, for a time. They say this loudly, and exaggerate it in their Eastern way. To them the English no longer appear as that superior race which beat them at Moodka, Ferozepore and Aliwal. From such a conviction to open hostility there is but a step with Eastern nations; a spark may kindle the blaze.

Altogether, the taking of Lucknow has no more put down the Indian insurrection than the taking of Delhi. This summer's campaign may produce such events that the British will have, next winter, to go substantially over the same ground again, and perhaps even to reconquer the Punjab. But in the best of cases, a long and harassing guerrilla warfare is before them—not an enviable thing for Europeans under an Indian sun.

June 15 1858—It is in this desultory warfare that the advantage of the sepoys lies. They can beat the English troops at marching to much the same extent that the English can beat them at fighting. An English column cannot move twenty miles a day; a sepoy force can move forty, and, if hard pushed, even sixty. It is this rapidity of movement which gives to the sepoy troops their chief value, and this, with their power of standing the climate and the comparative facility of feeding them, makes them indispensable in Indian warfare. The consumption of English troops in service, and especially in a summer campaign, is enormous. Already, the lack of men is severely felt. It may become necessary to chase the flying rebels from one end of India to the other. For that purpose, European troops

* Excerpts from K. Marx and F. Engels, articles in *New York Daily Tribune*, May 25, June 15, July 21, 1858. [Republished in Avinieri, ed., *Marx on Colonialism*, pp. 286, 299 f., 308 f., 328 f.]

would hardly answer, while the contact of the wandering rebels with the native regiments of Bombay and Madras, which have hitherto remained faithful, might lead to new revolts.

Even without any accession of new mutineers, there are still in the field not less than a hundred and fifty thousand armed men, while the unarmed population fail to afford the English either assistance or information.

July 21 1858.—The insurgent warfare now begins to take the character of that of the Bedouins of Algeria against the French; with the difference that the Hindoos are far from being so fanatical, and that they are not a nation of horsemen. This latter is important in a flat country of immense extent. There are plenty of Mohammedans among them who would make good irregular cavalry; still the principal cavalry nations of India have not joined the insurrection so far. The strength of their army is in the infantry, and that arm being unfit to meet the English in the field, becomes a drag in guerrilla warfare in the plain; for in such a country the sinew of desultory warfare is irregular cavalry. How far this want may be remedied during the compulsory holiday the English will have to take during the rains, we shall see. This holiday will, altogether, give the natives an opportunity of reorganizing and recruiting their forces. Besides the organization of cavalry, there are two more points of importance. As soon as the cold weather sets in, guerrilla warfare alone will not do. Centres of operation, stores, artillery, intrenched camps or towns, are required to keep the British busy until the cold season is over; otherwise the guerrilla warfare might be extinguished before the next summer gives it fresh life. Gwalior appears to be, among others, a favourable point, if the insurgents have really got hold of it. Secondly, the fate of the insurrection is dependent upon its being able to expand. If the dispersed columns cannot manage to cross from Rohilcund into Rajpootana and the Mahratta country; if the movement remains confined to the northern central district, then, no doubt, the next winter will suffice to disperse the bands, and to turn them into dacoits, which will soon be more hateful to the inhabitants than even the pale-faced invaders.

*IVB, 1d. Marx and Engels, 'The Moorish War of 1860'** Jan. 19 1860.—The Spaniards, with all the reinforcements received up to the 8th December, were from 35,000 to 40,000 strong, and 30,000 men might be available for offensive operations. With such a force, the conquest of Tetuan ought to be easy. There are certainly no good roads, and the provisions of the army must all be carried from Ceuta. But how did the French manage in Algiers, or the English in India? Besides, Spanish mules and cart-horses are not so spoiled by good roads in their own country as to refuse to march on Moorish ground. No matter what O'Donnell may say by way of apology, there can be no excuse for this continued inactivity. The Spaniards are as strong now as they can reasonably expect to be at any time in the campaign, unless unexpected reverses should bring on extraordinary exertions. The Moors, on the contrary, are daily getting stronger. The camp at Tetuan, under Hadji Abd Saleem, which furnished the bodies attacking the Spanish line on December 3, had been swelled to 10,000 already, beside the garrison of the town. Another camp, under Mulay Abbas, was at Tangiers, and reinforcements were arriving constantly from the interior. This consideration alone ought to have induced O'Donnell to advance as soon as the weather permitted it. He has had good weather, but he has not advanced. There can be no doubt that this is a sign of sheer irresolution, and that he has found the Moors less despicable enemies than he expected. There is no question that the latter have fought uncommonly well, and the great complaints arising from the Spanish camp of the advantages the ground in front of Ceuta gives to the Moors is a proof of it.

The Spaniards say that in brushwood and ravines the Moors are very formidable, and, besides, they know every inch of the ground; but that, as soon as they get into the plains, the solidity of the Spanish infantry will soon compel the Moorish irregulars to face about and run. This is a rather doubtful way of arguing in an epoch where three-fourths of the time spent in every battle is devoted to skirmishing in broken ground. If the Spaniards, after halting six weeks before Ceuta, do not know

* Excerpts from K. Marx and F. Engels, articles in *New York Daily Tribune*, Jan. 19 and March 17, 1860. [Republished in Avinieri, ed., *Marx on Colonialism*, pp. 377 ff., 383 f., 394–7.]

the ground as well as the Moors, so much the worse for them. That broken ground is more favorable to irregulars than a level plain, is clear enough. But even in broken ground, regular infantry ought to be vastly superior to irregulars. The modern system of skirmishing, with supports and reserves behind the extended chain, the regularity of the movements, the possibility of keeping the troops well in hand, and making them support each other and act all toward one common end—all this gives such superiority to regular troops over irregular bands, that in the ground best adapted for skirmishing, no irregulars ought to be able to stand against them, even if two to one. But here at Ceuta the proposition is reversed. The Spaniards have the superiority of numbers, and yet they dare not advance. The only conclusion is that the Spanish army do not understand skirmishing at all, and that thus their individual inferiority in this mode of fighting balances the advantages which their discipline and regular training ought to give them. In fact, there seems to be an uncommonly great deal of hand-to-hand fighting with yataghan and bayonet. The Moors, when the Spaniards are close enough, stop firing and rush upon them, sword in hand, in the same way as the Turks used to do, and this is certainly not very pleasant for young troops like the Spaniards. But the many engagements that have occurred ought to have made them familiar with the peculiarities of Moorish fighting and the proper mode to meet it; and when we see the commander still hesitate and remain in his defensive position, we cannot form a very high estimate of his army.

March 17 1860.—It is evident from this that both appliances and ideas in the Spanish army are of a very old-fashioned character. With a fleet of steamers and sailing transports always within sight, this march is perfectly ridiculous, and the men disabled during it by cholera and dysentery, were sacrificed to prejudice and incapacity. The road built by the engineers was no real communication with Ceuta, for it belonged to the Spaniards nowhere except where they happened to encamp. To the rear, the Moors might any day render it impracticable. To carry a message, or escort a convoy back to Ceuta, a division of 5,000 men at least was required. During the whole of the march, the communication with that place was carried on by the steamers alone. And with all that, the provisions accompanying the army were so insufficient that before twenty days had passed the army was on the point of starvation, and saved only by the stores from the fleet. Why, then, build the road at all? For the artillery? The Spaniards must have known for certain that the Moors had no field-artillery, and that their own rifled mountain guns were superior to anything the enemy could bring against them. Why, then, trail all this artillery along with them, if the whole of it could be carried by sea from Ceuta to San Martin (at the mouth of the Wahad el Jehu or Tetuan River) in a couple of hours? For any extremity, a single battery of field-guns might have accompanied the army, and the Spanish artillery must be very clumsy, if they could not march it over any ground in the world at the rate of five miles a day. . . .

This closes the first act of the campaign, and if the Emperor of Morocco is not too obstinate, it will very likely close the whole war. Still, the difficulties incurred hitherto by the Spaniards—difficulties increased by the system on which they have conducted the war—show that if Morocco holds out, Spain will find it a very severe piece of work. It is not the actual resistance of the Moorish irregulars—that never will defeat disciplined troops as long as they hold together and can be fed; it is the uncultivated nature of the country, the impossibility of conquering anything but the towns, and to draw supplies even from them; it is the necessity of dispersing the army in a great many small posts, which, after all, cannot suffice to keep open a regular communication between the conquered towns, and which cannot be victualed unless the greater part of the force be sent to escort the convoys of stores over roadless country, and across constantly reappearing clouds of Moorish skirmishers. It is well known what it was for the French, during the five or six years of their African conquest, to re-victual even Blidah and Medeah, not to speak of stations further from the coast. With the rapid wear and tear of European armies in that climate, six or twelve months of such a war will be no joke for a country like Spain. . . .

This much is certain: the Spaniards have much to learn yet in warfare before they can compel Morocco to peace, if Morocco holds out for a year.

*IVB, 1e. Engels, 'Guerrilla War in France'** In the course of the last six weeks, the character of the [Franco-Prussian] war has markedly changed. The regular armies of France have disappeared. The struggle is being carried on by recently mobilized troops whose inexperience makes them more or less irregular. Wherever they attempt to mass and fight in the open, they are easily defeated; but when they fight under the cover of villages and towns equipped with barricades and embrasures, it becomes evident that they are capable of offering serious resistance. They are encouraged to carry on this type of struggle, with night surprise attacks and other methods of guerrilla warfare, by proclamations and orders from the government, which also advises the population of the district in which they operate to give them every possible assistance.

If the enemy possessed sufficient troops to occupy the whole of the country, this resistance could be easily broken. But for this, up to the surrender of Metz, he has not had the strength. The ubiquitous 'four Uhlans' are no longer able to ride into a village or town outside their own lines, demanding absolute subjection to their orders, without incurring the risk of captivity or death. Requisitioning detachments have to be accompanied by escorting troops, and single companies or squadrons quartering in a village must guard against night attacks, and also, when they are on the march, against attacks from the rear. The German positions are surrounded by a belt of disputed territory, and it is just here that popular resistance makes itself felt most seriously.

In order to break this popular resistance, the Germans are resorting to a type of martial law that is as obsolete as it is barbaric. They act on the principle that any town or village in the defense of which one or more inhabitants have taken part, have fired on German troops or generally assisted the French—any such town or village is to be burnt down. Further, any man found carrying weapons, and not in their eyes a regular soldier, is to be summarily shot. When there is any suspicion that a considerable section of a town has been guilty of such a misdeed, all men capable of bearing arms are to be massacred forthwith. For the past six weeks this policy has been pitilessly carried out, and is still at this moment in full sway. One cannot

*** Excerpts from F. Engels, *Pall Mall Gazette*, Nov. 11 1870.**

open a single German newspaper without coming on half a dozen reports of such military executions; these are made to appear as a matter of course, as a simple process of military justice, carried out with salutary firmness by 'honest soldiers against cowardly assassins and robbers.' There is, of course, no disorder, no looting, no raping of women, no irregularity. Indeed no. Everything is done systematically, and by order. The condemned village is surrounded, the inhabitants driven out, the provisions confiscated, the houses set alight. The real or imaginary culprits are brought before a court martial, where a brief, final confession and half a dozen bullets are their certain lot.

It is no exaggeration to say that wherever the German flying columns march into the heart of France, their path is all too often marked with fire and blood. It is hardly sufficient, in their power to resurrect this spirit. It was at this time that nizable as soldiers are the equivalent of banditry, and must be put down with fire and sword. Such an argument might have been valid in the day of Louis XIV or Frederick II, when there was no kind of fighting other than that of regular armies. But ever since the American War of Independence and up to the American War of Secession, it has been the rule rather than the exception, for the people to take part in war. Wherever a people has allowed itself to be subjected for no other reason than that its armies have been incapable of offering resistance, it has earned general contempt as a nation of cowards; and wherever a people has energetically waged such irregular warfare, the invader soon found it impossible to carry through the obsolete law of blood and fire. The English in America, the French under Napoleon in Spain, and in 1848, the Austrians in Italy and Hungary, were very soon compelled to treat popular resistance as an entirely legitimate form of warfare. They were compelled to do so from the fear of reprisals against their own prisoners. . . .

Of all the armies in the world, the Prussian army should have been the last to revive these practices. In 1806, Prussia collapsed solely because nowhere in the country was there any sign of such a national spirit of resistance. After 1807, the reorganizers and the administrators of the army did everything in their power to ressurrect this spirit. It was at this time that Spain furnished a glorious example of how a nation can resist an invading army. The military leaders of Prussia all pointed to it as an example worthy of the emulation of their compatriots. Scharnhorst, Gneisenau, Clausewitz—all were of the same opinion. Gneisenau even went to Spain himself to take part in the struggle against Napoleon. The whole military system that was subsequently introduced in Prussia was an attempt to mobilize popular resistance against the enemy, insofar as this was possible at all in an absolute monarchy. Not only had every fit man to join the army and serve in the reserves (*Landwehr*) up to his 40th year; boys between 17 and 20 and men between 40 and 65 were also included in the *levée en masse*, or mass conscription, in the final reserves (*Landsturm*) whose function it was to rise in the rear and on the flanks of the enemy, to interfere with his movements, and to cut off his supplies and his couriers; they were expected to use any weapon they could lay their hands on and to employ without distinction all available measures to harry the invader—'the more effective the measure the better'; nor was 'any kind of uniform to be worn,' so that the men of the *Landsturm* might at any moment resume their character of civilians, thus remaining unrecognizable to the enemy.

This *Landsturm Order* of 1813, as the document in question was called—its author being no other than Scharnhorst, the organizer of the Prussian army—was drawn up in this spirit of irreconcilable national resistance, according to which all means are valid, and the most effective the best. At that time, however, all this was to be done by the Prussians against the French; when the French chose to behave in precisely the same manner toward the Prussians, it was quite another matter. What had become patriotism in one case became banditry and assassination in the other.

The fact is that the present Prussian government is ashamed of this old semi-revolutionary *Landsturm Order*, and by its actions in France seeks to erase it from memory. But the deliberate atrocities they themselves have committed in France will, instead, call it all the more to mind. The argument brought forward in favor of so despicable a method of waging war serves only as proof that, if the Prussian army has immeasurably improved since Jena, the Prussian government on the other hand, is ripening for the conditions that made Jena possible.

*IVB, 2. Lenin, 'On Guerrilla Action'**

Let us begin from the beginning. What are the fundamental demands which every Marxist should make of an examination of the question of forms of struggle? In the first place, Marxism differs from all primitive forms of socialism by not binding the movement to any one particular form of struggle. It recognizes the most varied forms of struggle; and it does not 'concoct' them, but only generalizes, organizes, gives conscious expression to those forms of struggle of the revolutionary classes which arise of themselves in the course of the movement. Absolutely hostile to all abstract formulas and to all doctrinaire recipes, Marxism demands an attentive attitude to the *mass* struggle in progress, which, as the movement develops, as the class-consciousness of the masses grows, as economic and political crises become acute, continually gives rise to new and more varied methods of defense and attack. Marxism, therefore, positively does not reject any form of struggle. Under no circumstances does Marxism confine itself to the forms of struggle possible and in existence at the given moment only, recognizing as it does that new forms of struggle, unknown to the participants of the given period, *inevitably* arise as the given social situation changes. In this respect Marxism *learns*, if we may so express it, from mass practice, and makes no claim whatever to *teach* the masses forms of struggle invented by 'systematizers' in the seclusion of their studies. We know—said Kautsky, for instance, when examining the forms of social revolution—that the coming crisis will introduce new forms of struggle that we are now unable to foresee.

In the second place, Marxism demands an absolutely *historical* examination of the question of the forms of struggle. To treat this question apart from the concrete historical situation betrays a failure to understand the rudiments of dialectical materialism. At different stages of economic evolution, depending on differences in political, national-cultural, living and other conditions, different forms of struggle come to the fore and become the principal forms of struggle; and in connection with this, the secondary, auxiliary forms of struggle undergo

* Excerpts from V. I. Lenin, 'On Guerrilla Action' (1906), *Collected Works*, XI: 213-23. [Originally published in *Proletary*, Sept. 30 1906.]

change in their turn. To attempt to answer yes or no to the question whether any particular means of struggle should be used, without making a detailed examination of the concrete situation of the given movement at the given stage of its development, means completely to abandon the Marxist position.

These are the two principal theoretical propositions by which we must be guided. The history of Marxism in Western Europe provides an infinite number of examples corroborating what has been said. European Social-Democracy at the present time regards parliamentarism and the trade union movement as the principal forms of struggle; it recognized insurrection in the past, and is quite prepared to recognize it, should conditions change, in the future—despite the opinion of bourgeois liberals like the Russian Cadets and the *Bezzaglavtsi*. Social-Democracy recognized street barricade fighting in the 40's, rejected it for definite reasons at the end of the 19th century, and expressed complete readiness to revise the latter view and to admit the expediency of barricade fighting, after the experience of Moscow, which, in the words of K. Kautsky, initiated new tactics of barricade fighting. . . .

The phenomenon in which we are interested is the *armed* struggle. It is conducted by individuals and by small groups. Some belong to revolutionary organizations, while others (the *majority* in certain parts of Russia) do not belong to any revolutionary organization. Armed struggle pursues two *different* aims, which must be *strictly* distinguished: in the first place, this struggle aims at assassinating individuals, chiefs and subordinates in the army and police; in the second place, it aims at the confiscation of monetary funds both from the government and from private persons. The confiscated funds go partly into the treasury of the party, partly for the special purpose of arming and preparing for an uprising, and partly for the maintenance of persons engaged in the struggle we are describing. The big expropriations go mostly, and sometimes entirely, to the maintenance of the 'expropriators.' This form of struggle undoubtedly became widely developed and extensive only in 1906, i.e., after the December uprising. The intensification of the political crisis to the point of an armed struggle and, in particular, the intensification of poverty, hunger and unemployment in town and country was one of the important causes of the struggle we are describing. This form of struggle was adopted as the preferable and even *exclusive* form of social struggle by the vagabond elements of the population, the *lumpen* proletariat and anarchist groups. Declaration of martial law, mobilization of fresh troops, Black-Hundred pogroms (Sedlets), and military courts must be regarded as the 'retaliatory' form of struggle adopted by the autocracy.

The usual appraisal of the struggle we are describing is that it is anarchism, Blanquism, the old terrorism, the acts of individuals isolated from the masses, which demoralize the workers, repel wide strata of the population, disorganize the movement and injure the revolution. Examples in support of this appraisal can easily be found in the events reported every day in the newspapers.

But are such examples convincing?. . . .

The old Russian terrorism was an affair of the intellectual conspirator; today as a general rule guerrilla warfare is waged by the worker combatant, or simply by the unemployed worker. Blanquism and anarchism easily occur to the minds of people who have a weakness for stereotype. . . . We must realize what forms of struggle inevitably arise under such circumstances, and not try to shirk the issue by a collection of words learned by rote, such as are used equally by the Cadets and the *Novoye Vremya*-ites: anarchism, robbery, hooliganism! . . . Guerrilla warfare is an inevitable form of struggle at a time when the mass movement has actually reached the point of an uprising and when fairly large intervals occur between the big 'engagements' in the civil war.

It is not guerrilla actions which disorganize the movement, but the weakness of a party which is incapable of taking such actions *under its control.* That is why the anathemas which we Russians usually hurl against guerrilla actions go hand in hand with secret, casual, unorganized guerrilla actions which really do disorganize the party. Being incapable of understanding what historical conditions give rise to this struggle, we are incapable of neutralizing its deleterious aspects. Yet the struggle is going on. It is engendered by powerful economic and political causes. It is not in our power to eliminate these causes or to eliminate this struggle. Our complaints against guerrilla warfare are complaints against our party weakness in the matter of an uprising.

What we have said about disorganization also applies to demoralization. It is not guerrilla warfare which demoralizes, but *unorganized* irregular, non-party guerrilla acts. We shall not rid ourselves one least bit of this *most unquestionable* demoralization by condemning and cursing guerrilla actions, for condemnation and curses are absolutely incapable of putting a stop to a phenomenon which has been engendered by profound economic and political causes. It may be objected that if we are incapable of putting a stop to an abnormal and demoralizing phenomenon, this is no reason why the *party* should adopt abnormal and demoralizing methods of struggle. But such an objection would be a purely bourgeois-liberal and not a Marxist objection, because a Marxist cannot regard civil war, or guerrilla warfare, which is one of its forms, as abnormal and demoralizing *in general.* A Marxist bases himself on the class struggle, and not social peace. In certain periods of acute economic and political crisis the class struggle ripens into a direct civil war, i.e., into an armed struggle between two sections of the people. In such periods a Marxist is *obliged* to take the stand of civil war. Any moral condemnation of civil war would be absolutely impermissible from the standpoint of Marxism. . . .

When I see Social-Democrats proudly and smugly declaring, 'we are not anarchists, thieves, robbers, we are superior to all this, we reject guerrilla warfare'—I ask myself: Do these people realize what they are saying? Armed clashes and conflicts between the Black-Hundred government and the population are taking place all over the country. This is an absolutely inevitable phenomenon at the present stage of development of the revolution. The population is spontaneously and in an unorganized way—and for that very reason often in unfortunate and *undesirable* forms—reacting to this phenomenon also by armed conflicts and attacks. I can understand us refraining from party leadership of *this* spontaneous struggle in a particular place or at a particular time because of the weakness and unpreparedness of our organization. I realize that this question must be settled by the local practical workers, and that the remolding of weak and unprepared organizations is no easy matter. But when I see a Social-Democratic theoretician or publicist not displaying regret over this unpreparedness, but rather a proud smugness and a self-exalted tendency to repeat phrases learned by rote in early youth about anarchism, Blanquism and terrorism, I am hurt by this degradation of the most revolutionary doctrine in the world.

It is said that guerrilla warfare brings the class-conscious proletarians into close association with degraded, drunken riff-raff. That is true. But it only means that the party of the proletariat can never regard guerrilla warfare as the only, or even as the chief, method of struggle; it means that this method must be subordinated to other methods, that this method must be commensurate with the chief methods of warfare, and must be ennobled by the enlightening and organizing influence of socialism. And without this *latter* condition, *all*, positively all, methods of struggle in bourgeois society bring the proletariat into close association with the various non-proletarian strata above and below it, and, if left to the spontaneous course of events, become frayed, corrupted and prostituted.

The forms of struggle in the Russian revolution are distinguished by their colossal variety compared with the bourgeois revolutions in Europe. Kautsky partly foretold this in 1902 when he said that the future revolution (with the exception *perhaps* of Russia, he added) might be not so much a struggle of the people against the government as a struggle between two sections of the people. In Russia we undoubtedly see a wider development of this *latter* struggle than in the bourgeois revolutions in the West. The enemies of our revolution among the people are few in number, but as the struggle grows more acute they become more and more organized and receive the support of the reactionary strata of the bourgeoisie. It is therefore absolutely natural and inevitable that in *such* a period, a period of nation-wide political strikes, an *uprising* cannot assume the old form of individual acts restricted to a very short time and to a very small area. It is absolutely natural and inevitable that the uprising should assume the higher and more complex form of a prolonged civil war embracing the whole country, i.e., an armed struggle between two sections of the people. Such a war cannot be conceived otherwise than as a series of a few big engagements at comparatively long intervals and a large number of small encounters during these intervals. That being so—and it is undoubtedly so—the Social-Democrats must absolutely make it their duty to create organizations best adapted to lead the masses in these big engagements and, as far as possible, in these small encounters as well. In a period when the class struggle has become accentuated to the point of civil war, Social-Democrats must make it their duty not only to participate but also to play the leading role in *this civil war.* The Social-Democrats must train and prepare their organizations to be really able to act as a *belligerent side* which does not miss a single opportunity of inflicting damage on the enemy's forces. . . .

We have not the slightest intention of foisting on practical workers any artificial form of struggle, or even of deciding from our armchair what part any particular form of guerrilla warfare should play in the general course of the civil war in Russia. We are far from the thought of regarding a concrete assessment of particular guerrilla actions as indicative of a *trend* in Social-Democracy. But we do regard it as our duty to help as far as possible to arrive at a correct *theoretical* assessment of the new forms of struggle engendered by practical life. We do regard it as our duty relentlessly to combat stereotypes and prejudices which hamper the class-conscious workers in correctly presenting a new and difficult problem and in correctly approaching its solution.

*IVB, 3. Trotsky, 'Guerrilla Warfare: Positionalism and Attack'**

We are told that the doctrine of the Red Army comprises of partisan actions in the enemy's rear and raids deep behind the front lines. But the first big raid was made by Mamontov, while Petlura was the leader of partisan formations. What does this mean? Just how does the doctrine of the Red Army happen to coincide with the doctrines of a Mamontov and a Petlura?

Some comrades have tried to reduce the doctrine of the Red Army to the use of hand-carts for transport. Inasmuch as

* Excerpts from L. Trotsky, 'Unified Military Doctrine' (1921), *Military Writings*, pp. 24–7, 34 ff.

we lack macadam roads and armored trucks, we shall of course use hand-carts for transportation, that's better than lugging a machinegun on one's back. But what has military doctrine to do with it? This is an absolutely incredible manner of posing the question. Our backwardness and lack of technical preparation can nowise provide material for military doctrine.

As touches maneuvering, let me point out that we are not the inventors of the maneuverist principle. Our enemies also made extensive use of it, owing to the fact that relatively small numbers of troops were deployed over enormous distances and because of the wretched means of communication. Much has been said here about the seizure of cities, points, and so on. Mamontov captured them from us, and we from him. This is in the very nature of civil warfare. In one and the same theater of war, we had our allies behind Mamontov, while in our midst were Mamontov's allies. Mamontov executed our agentry; we, his. An attempt is now made to build a doctrine on this. It is absurd.

Comrade Tukhachevsky sins in the sphere of overhasty generalization. In his opinion positional warfare is defunct. This is absolutely wrong. Should we continue to live in peace conditions for 5 or 10 years—which is not at all excluded—a new generation will have grown up; the nerve-wracking war moods under which we labor will have disappeared. A retardation of the revolution in the West would mean a breathing spell for the bourgeoisie. Technology is being restored by them as well as by us. We shall be enabled to move up larger and better equipped masses of troops; and with an army of greater mass and better armament there is produced a denser and more stabilized front. An explanation for our excessive maneuvering—which resulted time and again in our advancing 100 versts only in order to retreat 150 versts—is to be found in the fact that the army was so very thin and weak in relation to the given spaces; the armament was so inadequate that the outcome of battles was decided by factors of secondary nature. Why should we seek to hold on to this? What we need is to go beyond this stage of maneuvering which is only the obverse side of guerrilla warfare. I have often recalled that in the first period of the building of our army some comrades said that large formations were no longer needed; that the best thing for us would be a regiment of two or three battalions with artillery and cavalry—and this would comprise an independent unit. Expressed herein was the idea of primitive maneuvering. We have gone beyond this and any idealization of maneuvering would be dangerous in the extreme.

We are proffered a solution to the problem of offense and defence. We are told that our army must take the offensive. There is a great deal of confusion here, and I am afraid that Comrade Tukhachevsky supports in this connection those who are muddling and who say that our army must be an offensive army. Why? Since war is the continuation of politics by other means, therefore our politics should be offensive. But are they? What about Brest Litovsk? And what about our yesterday's declaration of readiness to recognize pre-war debts? It is a maneuver.

Only a daredevil cavalry man is of the opinion that one must always attack. Only a simpleton is of the opinion that a retreat is tantamount to doom. Attack and retreat can be integral parts of a maneuver, and may equally lead to victory. At the Third World Congress of the Communist International there was a whole tendency which insisted that a revolutionary epoch permits only of attack. This is greatest heresy. It is the most criminal heresy which has cost the German proletariat needless blood and didn't bring victory. Were this tactic to be followed in the future it would lead to the destruction of the German revolutionary movement. In a civil war it is necessary to maneuver. And since war is the continuation of politics by other means, how can we possibly say that military doctrine always demands the attack?

You cite the Great French Revolution and its army. But don't forget that the French were at the time the most cultured people of Europe—not only the most revolutionary but the most cultured and in point of technology, the most powerful, provided, of course, we discount England which was powerless to act on land. France could permit herself the luxury of offensive politics. But she crashed none the less. Although France did long march triumphantly across Europe, it all terminated in Waterloo and the restoration of the Bourbons. But we are among the most uncultured, the most backward peoples of Europe. Historical fate compelled us to accomplish the proletarian revolution in an encirclement of other peoples not yet seized by it. Wars lie ahead of us and we must teach our General Staff to appraise the situation correctly. Should we attack or retreat? Precisely here, knowledge of the most flexible and elastic kind is required; and it would be the most colossal blunder for us to impose upon the members of our General Staff the doctrine: Attack always! It is the strategy of adventurism and not revolutionary strategy. . . .

In building the Red Army we utilized Red Guard detachments as well as the old statutes as well as peasant *atamans* and former Czarist generals. This, of course, might be designated as the absence of 'unified doctrine' in the sphere of forming the army and its commanding staff. But such an appraisal would be pedantically banal. Assuredly, we did not take a dogmatic 'doctrine' as our starting point. We actually created the army from the historical material ready at hand, unifying all this work from the standpoint of a workers' state fighting to preserve, intrench and extend itself. Those who can't get along without the metaphysically compromised word doctrine, might say that in creating the Red Army, the armed power on a new class foundation, we thereby built a new military doctrine, inasmuch as despite the diversity of practical measures and the multiplicity of ways and means employed in our military construction, there could not be nor was there either empiricism, barren of ideas, or subjective arbitrariness in the entire work which from beginning to end was fused together by the unity of the class revolutionary goal, by the unity of the will directed to this end, by the unity of the Marxist method of orientation.

Attempts have been made and frequently repeated to take the actual work of building the Red Army as a premise for the proletarian 'military doctrine.' As far back as 1917 the absolute maneuverist principle was counterposed to the 'imperialist' principle of positional warfare. The organizational form of the army itself was declared to be subordinate to the revolutionary maneuverist strategy. The corps, the division, even the brigade were proclaimed to be units much too ponderous: The heralds of proletarian 'military doctrine' proposed to reduce the entire armed strength of the republic to individual combined detachments or regiments. In essence, this was the ideology of partisan warfare, only slicked up a bit. On the extreme 'left,' partisan warfare was openly defended. A holy war was declared against statutes, against the old statutes because they were the expression of an out-lived military doctrine; against the new—because they resembled the old too much. True enough, even at that time the adherents of the new doctrine not only failed to provide a draft of new statutes but they did not even present a single article submitting our statutes to any kind of serious principled or rational criticism. Our utilization of the old officers, all the more so their appointment to commanding posts, was proclaimed to be incompatible with the application of the revolutionary military doctrine. And so on and so forth.

As a matter of fact, the noisy innovators were themselves wholly captives of the old military doctrine: The only difference was that they sought to put a minus sign wherever previously there was a plus. All their independent thinking came down to just that. However, the actual work of creating the armed forces of the workers' state proceeded along an altogether different path. We tried—especially in the beginning—to make the greatest possible use of the habits, usages, knowledge and means retained from the past; and we were absolutely unconcerned about whether the new army would differ greatly from the old in the formally organizational and technical sense, or on the other hand, how much resemblance it would bear to the latter. We built the army with the human and technical material ready at hand, seeking always and everywhere to render secure the domination of the proletarian vanguard in the organization of the army, that is, in the army's personnel, its leading staff, its consciousness and in its moods. The institution of commissars is not some kind of dogma derived from Marxism. Neither is it an integral part of the proletarian 'military doctrine.' Under specific conditions it simply proved to be an indispensable instrument of proletarian control, proletarian leadership and political education of the army, and for this reason it acquired an enormous importance in the life of the armed forces of the Soviet Republic. The old commanding staff we combined with the new one; and only in this way were we able to achieve the necessary result: The army proved capable of fighting in the service of the working class. In its aims, in the class composition of its commander-commissar corps, in its spirit and its entire political morale, the Red Army differs radically from all other armies in the world and stands hostilely opposed to them.

IVB, 4. Mao, Guerrilla Strategy, and the Struggle against Li Li-san and the Left Opportunists

*a. 'Problems of Strategy in China's Revolutionary War'** The Chinese Communist Party has led and continues to lead the stirring, magnificent and victorious revolutionary war. This war is not only the banner of China's liberation, but has international revolutionary significance as well. The eyes of the revolutionary people the world over are upon us. In the new stage, the stage of the anti-Japanese national revolutionary war, we shall lead the Chinese revolution to its completion and exert a profound influence on the revolution in the East and in the whole world. Our revolutionary war has proved that we need a correct Marxist military line as well as a correct Marxist political line. Fifteen years of revolution and war have hammered out such political and military lines. We believe that from now on, in the new stage of the war, these lines will be further developed, filled out and enriched in new circumstances, so that we can attain our aim of defeating the national enemy. History tells us that correct political and military lines do not emerge and develop spontaneously and tranquilly, but only in the course of struggle. These lines must combat 'Left' opportunism on the one hand and Right opportunism on the other. Without combating and thoroughly overcoming these harmful tendencies which damage the revolution and the revolutionary war, it would be impossible to establish a correct line and win victory in this war. It is for this reason that I often refer to erroneous views in this pamphlet. . . .

People who do not admit, do not know, or do not want to know that China's revolutionary war has its own characteristics have equated the war waged by the Red Army against the Kuomintang forces with war in general or with the civil war in the Soviet Union. The experience of the civil war in the Soviet Union directed by Lenin and Stalin has a world-wide

* Excerpts from Mao Tse-tung, 'Problems of Strategy in China's Revolutionary War' (1936), *Selected Military Writings*, pp. 92 ff., 101 ff., 105 f., 111 ff., 119 f., 136 ff., 141 ff., 145 ff.

significance. All Communist Parties, including the Chinese Communist Party, regard this experience and its theoretical summing-up by Lenin and Stalin as their guide. But this does not mean that we should apply it mechanically to our own conditions. In many of its aspects China's revolutionary war has characteristics distinguishing it from the civil war in the Soviet Union. Of course it is wrong to take no account of these characteristics or deny their existence. This point has been fully borne out in our ten years of war.

Our enemy has made similar mistakes. He did not recognize that fighting against the Red Army required a different strategy and different tactics from those used in fighting other forces. Relying on his superiority in various respects, he took us lightly and stuck to his old methods of warfare. This was the case both before and during his fourth 'encirclement and suppression' campaign in 1933, with the result that he suffered a series of defeats. . . .

But when the enemy changed his military principles to suit operations against the Red Army, there appeared in our ranks a group of people who reverted to the 'old ways'. They urged a return to ways suited to the general run of things, refused to go into the specific circumstances of each case, rejected the experience gained in the Red Army's history of sanguinary battles, belittled the strength of imperialism and the Kuomintang as well as that of the Kuomintang army, and turned a blind eye to the new reactionary principles adopted by the enemy. As a result, all the revolutionary bases except the Shensi-Kansu border area were lost, the Red Army was reduced from 300,000 to a few tens of thousands, the membership of the Chinese Communist Party fell from 300,000 to a few tens of thousands, and the Party organizations in the Kuomintang areas were almost all destroyed. In short, we paid a severe penalty, which was historic in its significance. This group of people called themselves Marxist–Leninists, but actually they had not learned an iota of Marxism–Leninism. Lenin said that the most essential thing in Marxism, the living soul of Marxism, is the concrete analysis of concrete conditions. That was precisely the point these comrades of ours forgot. . . .

In the period of the Li Li-san line in 1930, Comrade Li Li-san failed to understand the protracted nature of China's civil war and for that reason did not perceive the law that in the course of this war there is repetition over a long period of 'encirclement and suppression' campaigns and of their defeat (by that time there had already been three in the Hunan-Kiangsi border area and two in Fukien). Hence, in an attempt to achieve rapid victory for the revolution, he ordered the Red Army, which was then still in its infancy, to attack Wuhan, and also ordered a nation-wide armed uprising. Thus he committed the error of 'Left' opportunism. . . .

The view that the Red Army should under no circumstances adopt defensive methods was directly related to this 'Left' opportunism, which denied the repetition of 'encirclement and suppression' campaigns, and it, too, was entirely erroneous. . . . The only entirely correct proposition is that a revolution or a revolutionary war is an offensive but also involves defence and retreat. To defend in order to attack, to retreat in order to advance, to move against the flanks in order to move against the front, and to take a roundabout route in order to get on to the direct route—this is inevitable in the process of development of many phenomena, especially military movements. . . . The 'Left' opportunism of 1931-34, which mechanically opposed the employment of defensive military measures, was nothing but infantile thinking.

When will the pattern of repeated 'encirclement and suppression' campaigns come to an end? In my opinion, if the civil war is prolonged, this repetition will cease when a fundamental change takes place in the balance of forces. It will cease when the Red Army has become stronger than the enemy. Then we shall be encircling and suppressing the enemy and he will be resorting to counter-campaigns, but political and military conditions will not allow him to attain the same position as that of the Red Army in its counter-campaigns. It can be definitely asserted that by then the pattern of repeated 'encirclement and suppression' campaigns will have largely, if not completely, come to an end. . . .

The military experts of the newer and rapidly developing imperialist countries, namely, Germany and Japan, trumpet the advantages of the strategic offensive and come out against the strategic defensive. This kind of military thinking is absolutely unsuited to China's revolutionary war. These military experts assert that a serious weakness of the defensive is that it shakes popular morale, instead of inspiring it. This applies to countries where class contradictions are acute and the war benefits only the reactionary ruling strata or the reactionary political groups in power. But our situation is different. With the slogan of defending the revolutionary base areas and defending China, we can rally the overwhelming majority of the people to fight with one heart and one mind, because we are the oppressed and the victims of aggression. It was also by using the form of the defensive that the Red Army of the Soviet Union defeated its enemies during the civil war. . . .

When Marx said that once an armed uprising is started there must not be a moment's pause in the attack, he meant that the masses, having taken the enemy unawares in an insurrection, must give the reactionary rulers no chance to retain or recover their political power, must seize this moment to beat the nation's reactionary ruling forces when they are unprepared, and must not rest content with the victories already won, underestimate the enemy, slacken their attacks or hesitate to press forward, and so let slip the opportunity of destroying the enemy, bringing failure to the revolution. This is correct. It does not mean, however, that when we are already locked in battle with an enemy who enjoys superiority, we revolutionaries should not adopt defensive measures even when we are hard pressed. Only a prize idiot would think in this way. . . . By May 1928, basic principles of guerrilla warfare, simple in nature and suited to the conditions of the time, had already been evolved, that is, the sixteen-character formula: 'The enemy advances, we retreat; the enemy camps, we harass; the enemy tires, we attack; the enemy retreats, we pursue.' This sixteen-character formulation of military principles was accepted by the Central Committee before the Li Li-san line. Later our operational principles were developed a step further. At the time of our first counter-campaign against 'encirclement and suppression' in the Kiangsi base area, the principle of 'luring the enemy in deep' was put forward, and moreover, successfully applied. . . .

But beginning from January 1932, after the publication of the Party's 'Resolution on the Struggle for the Victory of the Revolution First in One or More Provinces', which contained serious errors of principle, the 'Left' opportunists attacked these correct principles, finally abrogated the whole set and instituted a complete set of contrary 'new principles' or 'regular principles'. From then on, the old principles were no longer to be considered as regular but were to be rejected as 'guerrilla-ism'. The opposition to 'guerrilla-ism' reigned for three whole years. Its first stage was military adventurism, in the second it turned into military conservatism and, finally, in the third stage it became flightism. It was not until the Central Committee held the enlarged meeting of the Political Bureau at Tsunyi, Kweichow Province, in January 1935 that this wrong line was declared bankrupt and the correctness of the old line reaffirmed. But at what a cost!

Those comrades who vigorously opposed 'guerrilla-ism' argued along the following lines. It was wrong to lure the enemy in deep because we had to abandon so much territory. Although battles had been won in this way, was not the situation different now? Moreover, was it not better to defeat the enemy without abandoning territory? And was it not better still to defeat the enemy in his own areas, or on the borders between his areas and ours? The old practices had had nothing 'regular' about them and were methods used only by guerrillas. Now our own state had been established and our Red Army had become a regular army. Our fight against Chiang Kai-shek had become a war between two states, between two great armies. History should not repeat itself, and everything pertaining to 'guerrilla-ism' should be totally discarded. The new principles were 'completely Marxist', while the old had been created by guerrilla units in the mountains, and there was no Marxism in the mountains. The new principles were the antithesis of the old. They were: 'Pit one against ten, pit ten against a hundred, fight bravely and determinedly, and exploit victories by hot pursuit'; 'Attack on all fronts'; 'Seize key cities'; and 'Strike with two "fists" in two directions at the same time'. When the enemy attacked, the methods of dealing with him were: 'Engage the enemy outside the gates', 'Gain mastery by striking first', 'Don't let our pots and pans be smashed', 'Don't give up an inch of territory' and 'Divide the forces into six routes'. The war was 'the decisive battle between the road of revolution and the road of colonialism', a war of short swift thrusts, blockhouse warfare, war of attrition, 'protracted war'. There were, further, the policy of maintaining a large rear service organization and an absolutely centralized command. Finally there was a large-scale 'house-moving'. And anyone who did not accept these things was to be punished, labelled an opportunist, and so on and so forth.

Without a doubt these theories and practices were all wrong. They were nothing but subjectivism. Under favourable circumstances this subjectivism manifested itself in petty-bourgeois revolutionary fanaticism and impetuosity, but in times of adversity, as the situation worsened, it changed successively into desperate recklessness, conservatism and flightism. They were the theories and practices of hotheads and ignoramuses; they did not have the slightest flavour of Marxism about them; indeed they were anti-Marxist. . . .

Such seemingly revolutionary 'Left' opinions originate from the revolutionary impetuosity of the petty-bourgeois intellectuals as well as from the narrow conservatism of the peasant small producers. People holding such opinions look at problems only one-sidedly and are unable to take a comprehensive view of the situation as a whole; they are unwilling to link the interests of today with those of tomorrow or the interests of the part with those of the whole, but cling like grim death to the partial and the temporary. Certainly, we should cling tenaciously to the partial and the temporary when, in the concrete circumstances of the time, they are favourable—and especially when they are decisive—for the whole current situation and the whole period, or otherwise we shall become advocates of letting things slide and doing nothing about them. That is why a retreat must have a terminal point. We must not go by the short-sightedness of the small producer. We should learn the wisdom of the Bolsheviks. The naked eye is not enough, we must have the aid of the telescope and the microscope. The Marxist method is our telescope and microscope in political and military matters. . . .

The kind of concentration of forces we advocate does not mean the abandonment of people's guerrilla warfare. To abandon small-scale guerrilla warfare and 'concentrate every single rifle in the Red Army', as advocated by the Li Li-san line, has long since been proved wrong. Considering the revolutionary war as a whole, the operations of the people's guerrillas and those of the main forces of the Red Army complement each other like a man's right arm and left arm, and if we had only the main forces of the Red Army without the people's guerrillas, we would be like a warrior with only one arm. In concrete terms, and especially with regard to military operations, when we talk of the people in the base area as a factor, we mean that we have an armed people. That is the main reason why the enemy is afraid to approach our base area.

It is also necessary to employ Red Army detachments for operations in secondary directions; not all the forces of the Red Army should be concentrated. The kind of concentration we advocate is based on the principle of guaranteeing absolute or relative superiority on the battlefield. To cope with a strong enemy or to fight on a battlefield of vital importance, we must have an absolutely superior force; for instance, a force of 40,000 was concentrated to fight the 9,000 men under Chang Hui-tsan on December 30, 1930, in the first battle of our first counter-campaign. To cope with a weaker enemy or to fight on a battlefield of no great importance, a relatively superior force is sufficient; for instance, only some 10,000 Red Army men were employed to fight Liu Ho-ting's division of 7,000 men in Chienning on May 29, 1931, in the last battle of our second counter-campaign.

That is not to say we must have numerical superiority on every occasion. In certain circumstances, we may go into battle with a relatively or absolutely inferior force. Take the case of going into battle with a relatively inferior force when we have only a rather small Red Army force in a certain area (it is not that we have more troops and have not concentrated them). Then, in order to smash the attack of the stronger enemy in conditions where popular support, terrain and weather are greatly in our favour, it is of course necessary to concentrate the main part of our Red Army force for a surprise attack on a segment of one flank of the enemy while containing his centre and his other flank with guerrillas or small detachments, and in this way victory can be won. In our surprise attack on this segment of the enemy flank, the principle of using a superior force against an inferior force, of using the many to defeat the few, still applies. The same principle also applies when we go into battle with an absolutely inferior force, for example, when a guerrilla force makes a surprise attack on a large White army force, but is attacking only a small part of it. . . .

We use the few to defeat the many—this we say to the rulers of China as a whole. We use the many to defeat the few—this we say to each separate enemy force on the battlefield. That is no longer a secret, and in general the enemy is by now well acquainted with our way. However, he can neither prevent our victories nor avoid his own losses, because he does not know when and where we shall act. This we keep secret. The Red Army generally operates by surprise attacks. . . .

Mobile warfare or positional warfare? Our answer is mobile warfare. So long as we lack a large army or reserves of ammunition, and so long as there is only a single Red Army force to do the fighting in each base area, positional warfare is generally useless to us. For us, positional warfare is generally inapplicable in attack as well as in defence.

One of the outstanding characteristics of the Red Army's operations, which follows from the fact that the enemy is powerful while the Red Army is deficient in technical equipment, is the absence of fixed battle lines. . . .

In a revolutionary civil war, there cannot be fixed battle lines, which was also the case in the Soviet Union. The difference between the Soviet Army and ours is that its battle lines were not so fluid as ours. There cannot be absolutely fixed battle lines in any war, because the vicissitudes of victory and defeat, advance and retreat, preclude it. But relatively fixed battle lines are often to be found in the general run of wars. Exceptions occur only where an army faces a much stronger enemy, as is the case with the Chinese Red Army in its present stage. . . .

Guerrilla-ism has two aspects. One is irregularity, that is, decentralization, lack of uniformity, absence of strict discipline, and simple methods of work. These features stemmed from the Red Army's infancy, and some of them were just what was needed at the time. As the Red Army reaches a higher stage, we must gradually and consciously eliminate them so as to make the Red Army more centralized, more unified, more disciplined and more thorough in its work—

in short, more regular in character. In the directing of operations we should also gradually and consciously reduce such guerrilla characteristics as are no longer required at a higher stage. Refusal to make progress in this respect and obstinate adherence to the old stage are impermissible and harmful, and are detrimental to large-scale operations.

The other aspect of guerrilla-ism consists of the principle of mobile warfare, the guerrilla character of both strategic and tactical operations which is still necessary at present, the inevitable fluidity of our base areas, flexibility in planning the development of the base areas, and the rejection of premature regularization in building the Red Army. In this connection, it is equally impermissible, disadvantageous and harmful to our present operations to deny the facts of history, oppose the retention of what is useful, and rashly leave the present stage in order to rush blindly towards a 'new stage', which as yet is beyond reach and has no real significance.

We are now on the eve of a new stage with respect to the Red Army's technical equipment and organization. We must be prepared to go over to this new stage. Not to prepare ourselves would be wrong and harmful to our future warfare. In the future, when the technical and organizational conditions in the Red Army have changed and the building of the Red Army has entered a new stage, its operational directions and battle lines will become more stable; there will be more positional warfare; the fluidity of the war, of our territory and of our construction work will be greatly reduced and finally disappear; and we will no longer be handicapped by present limitations, such as the enemy's superiority and his strongly entrenched positions.

At present we oppose the wrong measures of the period of the domination of 'Left' opportunism on the one hand and on the other the revival of many of the irregular features which the Red Army had in its infancy but which are now unnecessary. . . .

Because the reactionary forces are very strong, revolutionary forces grow only gradually, and this fact determines the protracted nature of our war. Here impatience is harmful and advocacy of 'quick decision' incorrect. . . . The reverse is true of campaigns and battles—here the principle is not protractedness but quick decision. Quick decision is sought in campaigns and battles, and this is true at all times and in all countries. In a war as a whole, too, quick decision is sought at all times and in all countries, and a long drawn-out war is considered harmful. China's war, however, must be handled with the greatest patience and treated as a protracted war. During the period of the Li Li-san line, some people ridiculed our way of doing things as 'shadow-boxing tactics' (meaning our tactics of fighting many battles back and forth before going on to seize the big cities), and said that we would not see the victory of the revolution until our hair turned white. Such impatience was proved wrong long ago. But if their criticism had been applied not to strategy but to campaigns and battles, they would have been perfectly right. . . .

Campaign and battle plans should call for our maximum effort in concentration of troops, mobile warfare, and so on, so as to ensure the destruction of the enemy's effective strength on the interior lines (that is, in the base area) and the quick defeat of his 'encirclement and suppression' campaign, but where it is evident that the campaign cannot be terminated on our interior lines, we should employ the main Red Army force to break through the enemy's encirclement and switch to our exterior lines (that is, the enemy's interior lines) in order to defeat him there. Now that the enemy has developed his blockhouse warfare to a high degree, this will become our usual method of operation. . . .

For the Red Army which gets almost all its supplies from the enemy, war of annihilation is the basic policy. Only by annihilating the enemy's effective strength can we smash his 'encirclement and suppression' campaigns and expand our revolutionary base areas. Inflicting casualties is a means of annihilating the enemy, or otherwise there would be no sense to it. We incur losses ourselves in inflicting casualties on the enemy, but we replenish ourselves by annihilating his units, thereby not only making good our losses but adding to the strength of our army. A battle in which the enemy is routed is not basically decisive in a contest with a foe of great strength. A battle of annihilation, on the other hand, produces a great and immediate impact on any enemy. Injuring all of a man's ten fingers is not as effective as chopping off one, and routing ten enemy divisions is not as effective as annihilating one of them. . . .

In establishing our own war industry we must not allow ourselves to become dependent on it. Our basic policy is to rely on the war industries of the imperialist countries and of our domestic enemy. We have a claim on the output of the arsenals of London as well as of Hanyang, and, what is more, it is delivered to us by the enemy's transport corps. This is the sober truth, it is not a jest.

*IVB, 4b. Mao, 'The Establishment of Base Areas'** What, then, are these base areas? They are the strategic bases on which the guerrilla forces rely in performing their strategic tasks and achieving the object of preserving and expanding themselves and destroying and driving out the enemy. Without such strategic bases, there will be nothing to depend on in carrying out any of our strategic tasks or achieving the aim of the war. It is a characteristic of guerrilla warfare behind the enemy lines that it is fought without a rear, for the guerrilla forces are severed from the country's general rear. But guerrilla warfare could not last long or grow without base areas. The base areas, indeed, are its rear.

History knows many peasant wars of the 'roving rebel' type, but none of them ever succeeded. In the present age of advanced communications and technology, it would be all the more groundless to imagine that one can win victory by fighting in the manner of roving rebels. However, this roving-rebel idea still exists among impoverished peasants, and in the minds of guerrilla commanders it becomes the view that base areas are neither necessary nor important. Therefore, ridding the minds of guerrilla commanders of this idea is a prerequisite for deciding on a policy of establishing base areas. The question of whether or not to have base areas and of whether or not to regard them as important, in other words, the conflict between the idea of establishing base areas and that of fighting like roving rebels, arises in all guerrilla warfare, and, to a certain extent, our anti-Japanese guerrilla warfare is no exception. Therefore the struggle against the roving-rebel

* Excerpt from Mao Tse-tung, 'Problems of Strategy in Guerrilla War Against Japan' (May 1938), *Selected Military Writings*, pp. 167 f.

ideology is an inevitable process. Only when this ideology is thoroughly overcome and the policy of establishing base areas is initiated and applied will there be conditions favourable for the maintenance of guerrilla warfare over a long period.

*IVB, 4c. Mao, 'Avoiding Decisive Battles'** We should resolutely fight a decisive engagement in every campaign or battle in which we are sure of victory; we should avoid a decisive engagement in every campaign or battle in which we are not sure of victory; and we should absolutely avoid a strategically decisive engagement on which the fate of the whole nation is staked. . . . In the first and second stages of the war, which are marked by the enemy's strength and our weakness, the enemy's objective is to have us concentrate our main forces for a decisive engagement. Our objective is exactly the opposite. We want to choose conditions favourable to us, concentrate superior forces and fight decisive campaigns or battles only when we are sure of victory . . .we want to avoid decisive engagements under unfavourable conditions when we are not sure of victory. . . . As for fighting a strategically decisive engagement on which the fate of the whole nation is staked, we simply must not do so, as witness the recent withdrawal from Hsuchow. The enemy's plan for a 'quick decision' was thus foiled, and now he cannot help fighting a protracted war with us. These principles are impracticable in a country with a small territory, and hardly practicable in a country that is very backward politically. They are practicable in China because she is a big country and is in an era of progress. If strategically decisive engagements are avoided, then 'as long as the green mountains are there, one need not worry about firewood', for even though some of our territory may be lost, we shall still have plenty of room for manœuvre and thus be able to promote and await domestic progress, international support and the internal disintegration of the enemy; that is the best policy for us in the anti-Japanese war. Unable to endure the arduous trials of a protracted war and eager for an early triumph, the impetuous theorists of quick victory clamour

* Excerpts from Mao Tse-tung, 'On Protracted War' (1938), *Selected Military Writings*, pp. 254 ff.

for a strategically decisive engagement the moment the situation takes a slightly favourable turn. To do what they want would be to inflict incalculable damage on the entire war, spell finis to the protracted war, and land us in the enemy's deadly trap; actually, it would be the worst policy. Undoubtedly, if we are to avoid decisive engagements, we shall have to abandon territory, and we must have the courage to do so when (and only when) it becomes completely unavoidable. At such times we should not feel the slightest regret, for this policy of trading space for time is correct. History tells us how Russia made a courageous retreat to avoid a decisive engagement and then defeated Napoleon, the terror of his age. Today China should do likewise.

IVC. Guerrilla Warfare: The Marxist Strategy of the Twentieth Century?

*1. Trotsky, 'The Danger of Generalizing a Guerrilla Strategy'**

[Frunze] expresses the idea that future revolutionary wars will approximate civil wars in type, and for this reason will be maneuverist in character. But just which civil war is being referred to here? The reference is obviously to our civil war which took place under the specific conditons of our immense spaces, sparse population and poor means of communication. But the misfortune lies in this, that the theses posit some sort of abstract type of civil war, taking as their starting point the alleged fact that maneuverability flows from the class nature of the proletariat and not from the reciprocal relations between the theater of war and the density of troops. But, after all, in addition to our civil war, we know of still another and sufficiently large-scale example in France—the Paris Commune! In this instance the immediate task consisted in defending the fortified Parisian place of arms, from where alone any future offensive could have unfolded. What was the Commune in a military respect? It was the defense of the fortified Parisian region. Defense could and should have been active and flexible, but Paris had to be defended at all costs. To sacrifice Paris for the sake of a maneuver would have meant to cut down the

* Excerpts from L. Trotsky, 'Our Current Basic Miilitary Tasks' (1922), *Military Writings*, pp. 84 f., 103 ff.

revolution at its roots. The Communards were unable to defend Paris; the counter-revolution conquered Paris and slaughtered tens of thousands of workers. How than can I, proceeding from the experience of the steppes of the Don, the Kuban and Siberia, tell the Parisian worker: From your class nature there flows maneuverability. A generalization of this sort, hastily made, is no joking matter!

In the highly developed industrial countries with their dense populations, with their huge living centers, with their White Guard cadres prepared in advance, the civil war may assume—and in many cases will undoubtedly assume—a far less mobile, a far more compact character, that is, one approximating positional warfare. Generally speaking, there cannot even be talk of some sort of absolute positionalism, all the more so in a civil war. In question here is the reciprocal relation between the elements of maneuverability and of positionalism. And here it is possible to state with certainty that even in our supermaneuverist strategy during the civil war the element of positionalism did exist and in certain instances played an important role. There is no room whatever for doubt that *in the civil war in the West the element of positionalism will occupy a far more prominent place than in our civil war.* Let some one try to dispute this. In the civil war in the West the proletariat, owing to its greater numerical strength will play a far greater and more decisive role than in our country. From this alone it is clear how false it is to tie up maneuverability with proletarian class nature. Hungary, during its Soviet days, didn't have sufficient territory to be able to create an army by retreating and maneuvering; for this reason the revolution had to be surrendered to the enemy (interjection by Voroshilov: 'They can maneuver in a different way.'). Naturally, it is a wonderful idea that it is possible to maneuver 'in a different way,' that is, to include maneuvers within the framework of defending a given place of arms. But in such a case positionalism would already dominate over maneuverability. Up to a certain point maneuvers will play an auxiliary role during the defense of a given region which is the proletarian hearth of the civil war itself. But when we speak of the maneuverist strategy of civil war what we have in mind is the Russian example wherein we manipulated enormous distances and cities with a view to preserving our living forces and preparing a blow at the living forces of the enemy. During the days of the Commune the situation in France was such that the loss of Paris meant the doom of the revolution. In Soviet Hungary the arena of struggle was larger but it still remained very restricted. But even our arena of maneuverability is not unlimited. . . .

For the sake of illustration let us take England and let us try to imagine what will be, or more correctly, may be the character of a civil war in the British Isles. Naturally, we cannot prophesy. Naturally, events may unfold in an altogether different way, but it is nevertheless profitable to try to imagine the march of revolutionary events under the peculiar conditions of a highly developed capitalist country in an insular position.

The proletariat constitutes the overwhelming majority of the population in England. It has many conservative tendencies. It is hard to budge. But in return, once it starts moving and after it overcomes the first organized opposition of internal enemies its ascendancy on the islands will prove to be overwhelming owing to its overwhelming numbers. Does this mean that the bourgeoisie of Great Britain will not make the attempt with the assistance of Australia, Canada, the United States and others to overthrow the English proletariat? Of course it will. For this, it will attempt to retain the navy in its hands. The bourgeoisie will require the navy not only to institute a famine blockade but also for purposes of invasion raids. The French bourgeoisie will not refuse black regiments. The same fleet that now serves for the defense of the British Isles and for keeping them supplied uninterruptedly with necessities will become the instrument of attack upon these islands. Proletarian Great Britain will thus turn out to be a beleaguered naval fortress. There is no way of retreat from it, unless into the ocean. And we have presupposed that the ocean will remain in enemy hands. The civil war will consequently assume the character of the defense of an island against warships and invasion raids. I repeat this is no prophecy: events may unfold in a different way. But who will be so bold as to insist that the scheme of civil war outlined by me is impossible? It is quite possible and even probable. It would be a good thing for our strategists to ponder over this. They would then become completely convinced how unfounded it is to deduce maneuverability from the revolutionary nature of the proletariat. For all anyone knows, the English proletariat may find itself compelled to cover the shores of its islands with trenches, deep ribbons of barbed wire defences and positional artillery.

Models of civil war approximating our recent past, we ought to seek not in Europe of the future but in the past of the United States. It is unquestionable that the civil war in the United States in the 'sixties of the last century discloses many features in common with our civil war. Why? Because there, too, you had enormous spaces, a sparse population, inadequate means of communication. Cavalry raids played an enormous role there, too. It is a remarkable thing that there the initiative likewise came from the 'Whites,' that is from the Southern slaveowners who waged war against the bourgeois and petty-bourgeois democrats of the North. The Southerners possessed prairies, plantations, prairie pasture lands, good horses and were accustomed to riding horseback. The initial raids, thousands of versts in depth, were executed by them. Following their example, the Northerners created their own cavalry. The war was of a diffused, maneuverist character and terminated in the victory of the Northerners who defended the progressive tendencies of economic development against the Southern plantation slaveowners.

Comrade Tukhachevsky expressed himself in basic agreement with me, but made certain reservations the meaning of which is not clear to me. 'That Comrade Trotsky,' says Tukhachevsky, 'keeps pulling back by the coattails is a useful thing.' But this is useful, insofar as I am able to gather, only up to a certain point; for the very urge to create something new, in the sense of proletarian strategy and tactics, seems to Tukhachevsky an urge that is fruitful and progressive. Comrade Frunze, marching along the same line but going much further, cites Engels who wrote in the 'fifties that the conquest of power by the proletariat and the evolution of socialist society will create the premises for a new strategy. I also have no doubts that if a country with a developed socialist economy were compelled to wage war against a bourgeois country (as Engels visualized the situation in his mind) the picture of the socialist country's strategy would be one that is entirely different. But this provides no grounds whatever for attempts to suck out of one's thumb a 'proletarian strategy' for the USSR today. A new strategic word grows out of the urge to improve and fructify the practice of war and not at all out of the mere urge to say 'something new.'

*IVC, 2. Lin Piao, 'The Countryside versus the City'**

Comrade Mao Tse-tung's theory of and policies for people's war have creatively enriched and developed Marxism-Leninism. The Chinese people's victory in the anti-Japanese war was a victory for people's war, for Marxism–Leninism and the thought of Mao Tse-tung. . . .

Today, the U.S. imperialists are repeating on a worldwide scale the past actions of the Japanese imperialists in China and other parts of Asia. It has become an urgent necessity for the people in many countries to master and use people's war as a weapon against U.S. imperialism and its lackeys. In every conceivable way U.S. imperialism and its lackeys are trying to extinguish the revolutionary flames of people's war. The Khrushchev revisionists, fearing people's war like the plague, are heaping abuse on it. The two are colluding to prevent and sabotage people's war. In these circumstances, it is of vital practical importance to review the historical experience of the great victory of the people's war in China and to recapitulate Comrade Mao Tse-tung's theory of people's war. . . .

The Communist party of China and Comrade Mao Tse-tung were able to lead the Chinese people to victory in the War of Resistance Against Japan primarily because they formulated and applied a Marxist-Leninist line. . . .

There had long been two basic contradictions in China—the contradiction between imperialism and the Chinese nation, and the contradiction between feudalism and the masses of the people. For ten years before the outbreak of the War of Resistance, the Kuomintang reactionary clique, which represented the interests of imperialism, the big landlords and the big bourgeoisie, had waged civil war against the Communist

* Excerpts from Lin Piao, 'Long Live the Victory of the People's War' (1969), in Jay Mallin, ed., *Strategy for Conquest* (Coral Gables, Fla.: University of Miami Press, 1970), pp. 125–8, 135–9, 141 f., 148–52, 154, 158–61.

party of China and the Communist-led Workers' and Peasants' Red Army, which represented the interests of the Chinese people. In 1931, Japanese imperialism invaded and occupied northeastern China. Subsequently, and especially after 1935, it stepped up and expanded its aggression against China, penetrating deeper and deeper into our territory. As a result of its invasion, Japanese imperialism sharpened its contradiction with the Chinese nation to an extreme degree and brought about changes in class relations within China. To end the civil war and to unite against Japanese aggression became the pressing nationwide demand of the people. Changes of varying degrees also occurred in the political attitudes of the national bourgeoisie and the various factions within the Kuomintang. And the Sian Incident of 1936 was the best case in point. . . .

As the contradiction between China and Japan ascended and became the principal one, the contradiction between China and imperialist countries such as Britain and the United States descended to a secondary or subordinate position. The rift between Japan and the other imperialist countries had widened as a result of Japanese imperialism's attempt to turn China into its own exclusive colony. This rendered it possible for China to make use of these contradictions to isolate and oppose Japanese imperialism.

In the face of Japanese imperialist aggression, was the party to continue with the civil war and the Agrarian Revolution? Or was it to hold aloft the banner of national liberation, unite with all the forces that could be united to form a broad national united front and concentrate on fighting the Japanese aggressors? This was the problem sharply confronting our party.

The Communist party of China and Comrade Mao Tse-tung formulated the line of the Anti-Japanese National United Front on the basis of their analysis of the new situation. Holding aloft the banner of national liberation, our party issued a call for national unity and united resistance to Japanese imperialism, a call which won fervent support from the people of the whole country. Thanks to the common efforts of our party and of China's patriotic armies and people, the Kuomintang ruling clique was eventually compelled to stop the civil war, and a new situation with Kuomintang-Communist cooperation for joint resistance to Japan was brought about. . . .

The peasantry constituted more than eighty per cent of the entire population of semicolonial and semifeudal China. They were subjected to the threefold oppression and exploitation of imperialism, feudalism, and bureaucrat-capitalism, and they were eager for resistance against Japan and for revolution. It was essential to rely mainly on the peasants if the people's war was to be won.

But at the outset not all comrades in our party saw this point. The history of our party shows that in the period of the First Revolutionary Civil War, one of the major errors of the Right opportunists, represented by Chen Tu-hsiu, was their failure to recognize the importance of the peasant question and their opposition to arousing and arming the peasants. In the period of the Second Revolutionary Civil War, one of the major errors of the 'Left' opportunists, represented by Wang Ming was likewise their failure to recognize the importance of the peasant question. They did not realize that it was essential to undertake long-term and painstaking work among the peasants and establish revolutionary base areas in the countryside; they were under the illusion that they could rapidly seize the big cities and quickly win nationwide victory in the revolution. The errors of both the Right and the 'Left' opportunists brought serious setbacks and defeats to the Chinese revolution.

As far back as the period of the First Revolutionary Civil War, Comrade Mao Tse-tung had pointed out that the peasant question occupied an extremely important position in the Chinese revolution, that the bourgeois-democratic revolution against imperialism and feudalism was in essence a peasant revolution and that the basic task of the Chinese proletariat in the bourgeois-democratic revolution was to give leadership to the peasants' struggle. . . .

To rely on the peasants, build rural base areas, and use the countryside to encircle and finally capture the cities—such was the way to victory in the Chinese revolution.

Basing himself on the characteristics of the Chinese revolution, Comrade Mao Tse-tung pointed out the importance of building rural revolutionary base areas:

Since China's key cities have long been occupied by the powerful imperialists and their reactionary Chinese allies, it is imperative for the revolutionary ranks to turn the backward villages into advanced, consolidated base areas, into great military, political, economic, and cultural bastions of the revolution from which to fight their vicious enemies who are using the cities for attacks on the rural districts, and in this way gradually to achieve the complete victory of the revolution through protracted fighting; it is imperative for them to do so if they do not wish to compromise with imperialism and its lackeys but are determined to fight on, and if they intend to build up and temper their forces, and avoid decisive battles with a powerful enemy while their own strength is inadequate.

Experience in the period of the Second Revolutionary Civil War showed that, when this strategic concept of Comrade Mao Tse-tung's was applied, there was an immense growth in the revolutionary forces and one Red base area after another was built. Conversely, when it was violated and the nonsense of the 'Left' opportunists was applied, the revolutionary forces suffered severe damage, with losses of nearly 100 percent in the cities and ninety percent in the rural areas.

During the War of Resistance Against Japan, the Japanese imperialist forces occupied many of China's big cities and the main lines of communication, but owing to the shortage of troops they were unable to occupy the vast countryside, which remained the vulnerable sector of the enemy's rule. Consequently, the possibility of building rural base areas became even greater. Shortly after the beginning of the War of Resistance, when the Japanese forces surged into China's hinterland and the Kuomintang forces crumbled and fled in one defeat after another, the Eighth Route and New Fourth armies, led by our party, followed the wise policy laid down by Comrade Mao Tse-tung and boldly drove into the areas behind the enemy lines in small contingents and established base areas throughout the countryside. . . .

In the anti-Japanese base areas, we carried out democratic reforms, improved the livelihood of the people, and mobilized and organized the peasant masses. Organs of anti-Japanese democratic political power were established on an extensive scale and the masses of the people enjoyed the democratic right to run their own affairs; at the same time we carried out the policies of 'a reasonable burden' and 'the reduction of rent and interest,' which weakened the feudal system of exploitation and improved the people's livelihood. As a result, the enthusiasm of the peasant masses was deeply aroused, while the various anti-Japanese strata were given due consideration and were thus united. In formulating our policies for the base areas, we also took care that these policies should facilitate our work in the enemy-occupied areas.

In the enemy-occupied cities and villages, we combined legal with illegal struggle, united the basic masses and all patriots, and divided and disintegrated the political power of the enemy and his puppets so as to prepare ourselves to attack the enemy from within in coordination with operations from without when conditions were ripe.

The base areas established by our party became the centre of gravity in the Chinese people's struggle to resist Japan and save the country. Relying on these bases, our party expanded and strengthened the people's revolutionary forces, persevered in the protracted war, and eventually won the War of Resistance Against Japan. . . .

At the same time, the work of building the revolutionary base areas was a grand rehearsal in preparation for nationwide victory. In these base areas, we built the party, ran the organs of state power, built the people's armed forces and set up mass organizations; we engaged in industry and agriculture and operated cultural, educational, and all other undertakings necessary for the independent existence of a separate region. Our base areas were in fact a state in miniature. And with the steady expansion of our work in the base areas, our party established a powerful people's army, trained cadres for various kinds of work, accumulated experience in many fields, and built up both the material and the moral strength that provided favorable conditions for nationwide victory.

The revolutionary base areas established in the War of Resistance later became the springboards for the People's War of Liberation, in which the Chinese people defeated the Kuomintang reactionaries. In the War of Liberation we continued the policy of first encircling the cities from the countryside and then capturing the cities, and thus won nationwide victory.

'Without a people's army the people have nothing.' This is the conclusion drawn by Comrade Mao Tse-tung from the Chinese people's experience in their long years of revolutionary struggle, experience that was bought in blood. This is a universal truth of Marxism–Leninism.

The special feature of the Chinese revolution was armed revolution against armed counterrevolution. The main form of struggle was war and the main form of organization was the army which was under the absolute leadership of the Chinese Communist Party, while all the other forms of organization and struggle led by our party were coordinated, directly or indirectly, with the war. . . .

The essence of Comrade Mao Tse-tung's theory of army building is that in building a people's army prominence must be given to politics, i.e., the army must first and foremost be built on a political basis. Politics is the commander, politics is the soul of everything. Political work is the lifeline of our army. True, a people's army must pay attention to the constant improvement of its weapons and equipment and its military technique, but in its fighting it does not rely purely on weapons and technique, it relies mainly on politics, on the proletarian revolutionary consciousness and courage of the commanders and fighters, on the support and backing of the masses.

Owing to the application of Comrade Mao Tse-tung's line on army building, there has prevailed in our army at all times a high level of proletarian political consciousness, an atmosphere of keenness to study the thought of Mao Tse-tung, an excellent morale, a solid unity and a deep hatred for the enemy, and thus a gigantic moral force has been brought into being. In battle it has feared neither hardships nor death, it has been able to charge or hold its ground as the conditions require. One man can play the role of several, dozens, or even hundreds, and miracles can be performed.

All this makes the people's army led by the Chinese Communist Party fundamentally different from any bourgeois army, and from all the armies of the old type which served the exploiting classes and were driven and utilized by a handful of people. The experience of the people's war in China shows that a people's army created in accordance with Comrade Mao Tse-tung's theory of army building is incomparably strong and invincible. . . .

Comrade Mao Tse-tung's great merit lies in the fact that he

has succeeded in integrating the universal truth of Marxism–Leninism with the concrete practice of the Chinese revolution and has enriched and developed Marxism–Leninism by his masterly generalization and summation of the experience gained during the Chinese people's protracted revolutionary struggle.

Comrade Mao Tse-tung's theory of people's war has been proved by the long practice of the Chinese revolution to be in accord with the objective laws of such wars and to be invincible. It has not only been valid for China, it is a great contribution to the revolutionary struggles of the oppressed nations and peoples throughout the world. . . .

In the last analysis, the Marxist–Leninist theory of proletarian revolution is the theory of the seizure of state power by revolutionary violence, the theory of countering war against the people by people's war. As Marx so aptly put it, 'Force is the midwife of every old society pregnant with a new one.'

It was on the basis of the lessons derived from the people's wars in China that Comrade Mao Tse-tung, using the simplest and the most vivid language, advanced the famous thesis that 'political power grows out of the barrel of a gun.'

He clearly pointed out:

> The seizure of power by armed force, the settlement of the issue by war, is the central task and the highest form of revolution. This Marxist-Leninist principle of revolution holds good universally, for China and for all other countries.

War is the product of imperialism and the system of exploitation of man by man. Lenin said that 'war is always and everywhere begun by the exploiters themselves, by the ruling and oppressing classes.' So long as imperialism and the system of exploitation of man by man exist, the imperialists and reactionaries will invariably rely on armed force to maintain their reactionary rule and impose war on the oppressed nations and peoples. This is an objective law independent of man's will. . . .

The history of people's war in China and other countries provides conclusive evidence that the growth of the people's revolutionary forces from weak and small beginnings into strong and large forces is a universal law of development of class struggle, a universal law of development of people's war.

A people's war inevitably meets with many difficulties, with ups and downs and setbacks in the course of its development, but no force can alter its general trend towards inevitable triumph. . . .

Dialectical and historical materialism teaches us that what is important primarily is not that which at the given moment seems to be durable and yet is already beginning to die away, but that which is arising and developing, even though at the given moment it may not appear to be durable, for only that which is arising and developing is invincible.

Why can the apparently weak new-born forces always triumph over the decadent forces which appear so powerful? The reason is that truth is on their side and that the masses are on their side, while the reactionary classes are always divorced from the masses and set themselves against the masses.

This has been borne out by the victory of the Chinese revolution, by the history of all revolutions, the whole history of class struggle and the entire history of mankind.

The imperialists are extremely afraid of Comrade Mao Tse-tung's thesis that 'imperialism and all reactionaries are paper tigers,' and the revisionists are extremely hostile to it. They all oppose and attack this thesis and the philistines follow suit by ridiculing it. But all this cannot in the least diminish its importance. The light of truth cannot be dimmed by anybody. . . .

It must be emphasized that Comrade Mao Tse-tung's theory of the establishment of rural revolutionary base areas and the encirclement of the cities from the countryside is of outstanding and universal practical importance for the present revolutionary struggles of all the oppressed nations and peoples, and particularly for the revolutionary struggles of the oppressed nations and peoples in Asia, Africa, and Latin America against imperialism and its lackeys.

Many countries and peoples in Asia, Africa, and Latin America are now being subjected to aggression and enslavement on a serious scale by the imperialists headed by the United States and their lackeys. The basic political and economic conditions in many of these countries have many similarities to those that prevailed in old China. As in China, the peasant question is extremely important in these regions. The peasants constitute the main force of the national-democratic revolution against the imperialists and their lackeys. In committing aggression against these countries, the imperialists usually begin by seizing the big cities and the main lines of communication, but they are unable to bring the vast countryside completely under their control. The countryside, and the countryside alone, can provide the broad areas in which the revolutionaries can maneuver freely. The countryside, and the countryside alone, can provide the revolutionary bases from which the revolutionaries can go forward to final victory. Precisely for this reason, Comrade Mao Tse-tung's theory of establishing revolutionary base areas in the rural districts and encircling the cities from the countryside is attracting more and more attention among the people in these regions.

Taking the entire globe, if North America and Western Europe can be called 'the cities of the world,' then Asia, Africa, and Latin America constitute 'the rural areas of the world.' Since World War II, the proletarian revolutionary movement has for various reasons been temporarily held back in the North American and Western European capitalist countries, while the people's revolutionary movement in Asia, Africa, and Latin America has been growing vigorously. In a sense, the contemporary world revolution also presents a picture of the encirclement of cities by the rural areas. In the final analysis, the whole cause of world revolution hinges on the revolutionary struggles of the Asian, African, and Latin American peoples who make up the overwhelming majority of the world's population. . . .

Mao Tse-tung's thought has been the guide to the victory of the Chinese revolution. It has integrated the universal truth of Marxism-Leninism with the concrete practice of the Chinese revolution and creatively developed Marxism–Leninism, thus adding new weapons to the arsenal of Marxism–Leninism.

Ours is the epoch in which world capitalism and imperialism are heading for their doom and socialism and communism are marching to victory. Comrade Mao Tse-tung's theory of people's war is not only a product of the Chinese revolution, but has also the characteristics of our epoch. The new experience gained in the people's revolutionary struggles in various countries since World War II has provided continuous evidence that Mao Tse-tung's thought is a common asset of the revolutionary people of the whole world. This is the great international significance of the thought of Mao Tse-tung.

*IVC, 3. Régis Debray, 'Guerrilla War and the Military Vanguard of the Revolution'**

One may well consider it a stroke of good luck that Fidel had not read the military writings of Mao Tse-tung before disembarking on the coast of Oriente: he could thus invent, on the spot and out of his own experience, principles of a military doctrine in conformity with the terrain. It was only at the end of the war, when their tactics were already defined, that the rebels discovered the writings of Mao. But once again in Latin America, militants are reading Fidel's speeches and Che Guevara's writings with eyes that have already read Mao on the anti-Japanese war, Giap, and certain texts of Lenin—and they think they recognize the latter in the former. Classical visual superimposition, but dangerous, since the Latin American revolutionary war possesses highly special and profoundly distinct conditions of development, which can only be discovered through a particular experience. In that sense, all the theoretical works on people's war do as much harm as good. They have been called the grammar books of the war. But a foreign language is learned faster in a country where it must be spoken than at home studying a language manual. In time of war questions of speed are vital, especially in the early stages when an unarmed and inexperienced guerrilla band must confront a well-armed and knowledgeable enemy.

Fidel once blamed certain failures of the guerrillas on a purely intellectual attitude toward war. The reason is understandable: aside from his physical weakness and lack of adjustment to rural life, the intellectual will try to grasp the present through preconceived ideological constructs and live it through books. He will be less able than others to invent, improvise, make do with available resources, decide instantly on bold moves when he is in a tight spot. Thinking that he already knows, he will learn more slowly, display less flexibility. And

*Excerpts from Régis Debray, *Revolution in the Revolution?* (New York: Monthly Review Press, 1967), pp. 20 f., 28 f., 33 f., 60, 62 f., 88-91, 96-9, 102 f., 105 ff., 109 ff., 113 f., 121 f.

the irony of history has willed, by virtue of the social situation of many Latin American countries, the assignment of precisely this vanguard role to students and revolutionary intellectuals, who have had to unleash, or rather initiate, the highest forms of class struggle. . . .

In the ideological background of self-defense there are to be found ideologies which Lenin repeatedly described as indigenous to the working class and which he said would again and again come to the fore whenever Marxists and Communists lowered their guard: 'economism' and 'spontaneity.'. . .

Self-defense does not suffer from a lack of boldness among its promoters. Quite to the contrary, it frequently suffers from a profusion of admirable sacrifices, of wasted heroism leading nowhere—that is, leading anywhere except to the conquest of political power. It is therefore better to speak of armed spontaneity. Its very ideological origin reveals to us the epoch in which it was born: prior to Marx. . . .

In short, there were workers' insurrections before the advent of scientific socialism, as there were peasant wars before there were revolutionary guerrilla wars. But neither in the one case nor in the other is there an interrelation. Guerrilla warfare is to peasant uprisings what Marx is to Sorel.

Just as economism denies the vanguard role of the party, self-defense denies the role of the armed unit, which is organically separate from the civilian population. Just as reformism aims to constitute a mass party without selection of its militants or disciplined organization, self-defense aspires to integrate everyone into the armed struggle, to create a mass guerrilla force, with women, children, and domestic animals in the midst of the guerrilla column. . . .

Let us for the moment decide to take the [present-day Latin American] Trotskyist conception seriously, and not as the pure and simple provocation that it is in practice. We will observe a certain amount of confusion. First, the imposition of the working-class model of factory cells and proletarian trade unions on the peasant reality (what is valid for a factory or capitalist metropolis is valid for the Indian community, which dates back to Mayan or Inca society); the underestimation, paradoxical after such an imposition, of the role of the working class as the leading force of the revolution; the confusing of armed struggle—as a long process of building up a popular army in the field—with a direct assault on power or a Bolshevik-type insurrection in the city; a total incomprehension of the relation of forces between the peasantry and the ruling class. Whatever the theoretical confusions, and there are many, one thing is certain: this beautiful verbal apparatus operates in reality like a trap, and the trap shuts on the agricultural workers and sometimes on the organizers as well. To promote public assemblies of the people in an Indian village, or open union meetings, is simply to denounce the inhabitants to the forces of repression and the political cadres to the police: it is to send them to prison or to their graves. . . .

At bottom Trotskyism is a metaphysic paved with good intentions. It is based on a belief in the natural goodness of the workers, which is always perverted by evil bureaucracies but never destroyed. There is a proletarian essence within peasants and workers alike which cannot be altered by circumstances. For them to become aware of it themselves, it is only necessary that they be given the word, that objectives be set for them which they see without seeing and which they know without knowing. Result: socialism becomes a reality, all at once, without delay, neat and tidy.

Because Trotskyism, in its final state of degeneration, is a medieval metaphysic, it is subject to the monotonies of its function. In space—everywhere the same: the same analyses and perspectives serve equally well for Peru and Belgium. In time—immutable: Trotskyism has nothing to learn from history. It already has the key to it: the proletariat, essentially wholesome and unfailingly socialist—eternally at odds, in its union activity, with the perverse formalism of the Stalinist bureaucracies. Prometheus struggling ceaselessly against a Zeus of a thousand disguises in order to steal from him the fire of liberation and keep it burning. Has anyone ever seen a concrete analysis of a concrete situation from the pen of a Trotskyist?...

That an intellectual, especially if he is a bourgeois, should speak of strategy before all else, is normal. Unfortunately, however, the right road, the only feasible one, sets out from tactical data, rising gradually toward the definition of strategy. The abuse of strategy and the lack of tactics is a delightful vice, characteristic of the contemplative man—a vice to which we, by writing these lines, must also plead guilty. All the more reason to remain aware of the *inversion* of which we are victims when we read theoretical works. They present to us in the form of principles and a rigid framework certain so-called strategic concepts which in reality are the result of a series of experiments of a tactical nature. Thus it is that we take a result for a point of departure. For a revolutionary group, military strategy springs first of all from a combination of political and social circumstances, from its own relationship with the population, from the limitations of the terrain, from the opposing forces and their weaponry, etc. Only when these details have been mastered can serious plans be made. Finally—and this is even truer for guerrilla forces than for regular armies—there are no details in the action or, if you prefer, everything is a matter of detail.

This slow climb from tactics to surrounding and corresponding strategy, along with the experience gained at all intermediate stages, is to some extent the history of the Cuban Revolution. . . . For the guerrilla force to attempt to occupy a fixed base or to depend on a security zone, even one of several thousand square kilometers in area, is, to all appearances, to deprive itself of its best weapon, mobility, to permit itself to be contained within a zone of operations, and to allow the enemy to use its most effective weapons. The notion of the security zone raised to a fetish is the fixed encampment set up in reputedly inaccessible spots. This reliance on the characteristics of the terrain alone is always dangerous; after all, no place is inaccessible; if anyone has been able to reach it, then so can the enemy. The rule of conduct observed by the Rebel Army from the beginning was to operate as if the enemy always knew where the guerrilla force was and as if an attack would be mounted from the nearest military post. The struggle against infiltration and betrayal in Cuba thus tended to take the form of extreme mobility. Since every individual who left an encampment was considered to be a potential source of betrayal, voluntary or forced, camp sites were unavoidably temporary and subject to constant shifting, during the first stage. . . .

'Technicism' and 'militarism'—are these terms not justly applied to those who label as technicism and militarism the wish to encompass all forms of struggle within the context of guerrilla warfare, to those who counterpose political line to military strategy, political leadership to military leadership? They live in a double world, genuinely dualist and—why not say it?—deriving from a strongly *idealist* tradition: politics on one side, the military on the other. The people's war is considered to be a technique, practiced in the countryside and subordinated to the political line, which is conceived of as a super-technique, 'purely' theoretical, 'purely' political. Heaven governs the earth, the soul governs the body, the head governs the hand. The Word precedes the Act. The secular substitutes for the Word—talk, palaver, chatter—precede and regulate military activity, from the heavens above.

First, one cannot see how a political leadership, in the Latin America of today, can remain aloof from technical problems of war; it is equally inconceivable that there can be political cadres who are not simultaneously military cadres. It is the situation itself, present and future, that requires this: 'the cadres' of the mass armed struggle will be those who participate in it and who, in the field, prove their ability as its leaders. But how many political leaders prefer to concern themselves, day after day, with world trade unionism or to involve themselves in the mechanisms of a thousand and one 'international democratic organizations' dedicated to their own survival rather than devote themselves to a serious and concrete study of military questions related to the war of their people? Furthermore, military technique assumes a special importance in Latin America. Unlike China, and Asia in general, the initially great disproportion between the strength of the revolutionary forces and that of the entire repressive mechanism, and the demographic consequences of poverty in the rural areas do not permit the immediate replacement of arms and technique by sheer mass and number of combatants. On the contrary, to compensate for this initial disproportion and for the relative demographic poverty of many countries, technique must be wielded with expertise. Whence the more important role here than elsewhere of, for example, mines, explosives, bazookas, modern automatic weapons, etc. In an ambush, for example, when the smallest detail and every minute count, the intelligent use of modern automatic arms, their firing plan, a coordinated program of fire can all compensate for the lack or scarcity of manpower on the revolutionary side. In a limited and defined number of seconds, three men can now liquidate a troop transport truck carrying thirty soldiers, whereas with the older type of guns, an equal number of *guerrilleros* would have been required. For the same reason the number one objective of a guerrilla group is to capture the arms of the enemy, not to attempt to annihilate it, unless necessary in order to take possession of its weapons. In brief, no detail is too small for a political-military chief: everything rests on details—on a single detail—and he himself must supervise them all.

Second, it has been proved that for the training of revolutionary cadres, the people's war is more decisive than political activity without guerrilla experience. Leaders of vision in Latin America today are young, lacking in long political experience prior to joining up with the guerrillas. It is ridiculous to continue to oppose 'political cadres' to 'military cadres,' 'political leadership' to 'military leadership.' Pure 'politicians'—who want to remain pure—cannot lead the armed struggle of the people; pure 'military men' can do so, and by the experience acquired in leading a guerrilla group, they become 'politicians' as well. . . . 'To those who show military ability, also give political responsibility.' It was worth the risk: Raúl Castro, Che Guevara, Camilo Cienfuegos, and scores of officers, who are today in the political leadership of a proletarian and peasant revolution.

But, there is a fact that we must not hide: The parties or organizations whose political leaderships have operated in this fashion—controlling their embryonic army from the outside, maintaining a duality of organization, removing their activists from the guerrilla force and sending them elsewhere for political training—are basing themselves on hallowed principles of organization, apparently essential to Marxist theory, that is, on a distinction between the military and the political. . . . Are we not repudiating by implication a hallowed principle, that of the distinctiveness of the party and its predominance over the people's army in the phase preceding the seizure of power, on the fallacious pretext that the principle is badly applied? Or is the principle itself not valid for all latitudes? Let us examine the problem at its root.

Now then, ['theoretical orthodoxy' insists] a class is

represented by a political party, not by a military instrumentality. The proletariat is represented by that party which expresses its class ideology, Marxism–Leninism. Only the leadership of this party can scientifically defend its class interests. . . . In brief, the party determines the political content and the goal to be pursued, and the people's army is merely an *instrument* of implementation. To take the popular army for the party would be to take the instrument for the goal, the means for the end: a confusion proper to technocracy—hence the terms 'technicism' and 'militarism' given to this deviation. . . .

In Cuba, military (operational) and political leadership have been combined on one man: Fidel Castro. Is this the result of mere chance, without significance, or is it an indication of an historically different situation? Is it an exception or does it foreshadow something fundamental? What light does it throw on the current Latin American experience? We must decipher this experience in time, and we must not rush to condemn history in the making because it does not conform to received principles. Fidel Castro said recently:

> I am accused of heresy. It is said that I am a heretic within the camp of Marxism–Leninism. Hmm! It is amusing that so-called Marxist organizations, which fight like cats and dogs in their dispute over possession of revolutionary truth, accuse us of wanting to apply the Cuban formula mechanically. They reproach us with a lack of understanding of the Party's role; they reproach us as heretics within the camp of Marxism–Leninism. . . .

Fidel Castro says simply that there is no revolution without a vanguard; that this vanguard is not necessarily the Marxist-Leninist party; and that those who want to make the revolution have the right and the duty to constitute themselves a vanguard, independently of these parties.

It takes courage to state the facts out loud when these facts contradict a tradition. There is, then, no metaphysical equation in which vanguard = Marxist–Leninist party; there are merely dialectical conjunctions between a given function—that of the vanguard in history—and a given form of organization—that of the Marxist-Leninist party. These conjunctions arise out of prior history and depend on it. Parties exist here on earth and are subject to the rigors of terrestrial dialectics.

If they have been born, they can die and be reborn in other forms. How does this rebirth come about? Under what form can the historic vanguard reappear? . . .

In Latin America, wherever armed struggle is on the order of the day, there is a close tie between biology and ideology. However absurd or shocking this relationship may seem, it is nonetheless a decisive one. An elderly man, accustomed to city living, molded by other circumstances and goals, will not easily adjust himself to the mountain nor—though this is less so—to underground activity in the cities. In addition to the moral factor—conviction—physical fitness is the most basic of all skills needed for waging guerrilla war; the two factors go hand in hand. A perfect Marxist education is not, at the outset, an imperative condition. That an elderly man should be proven militant—and possess a revolutionary training—is not, alas, sufficient for coping with guerrilla existence, especially in the early stages. Physical aptitude is the prerequisite for all other aptitudes; a minor point of limited theoretical appeal, but the armed struggle appears to have a rationale of which theory knows nothing.

A new organization. The reconstitution of the Party into an effective directive organism, equal to the historic task, requires that an end be put to the plethora of commissions, secretariats, congresses, conferences, plenary sessions, meetings, and assemblies at all levels—national, provincial, regional, and local. Faced with a state of emergency and a militarily organized enemy, such a mechanism is paralyzing at best, catastrophic at worst. It is the cause of the vice of excessive deliberation which Fidel has spoken of and which hampers executive, centralized, and vertical methods, combined with the large measure of tactical independence of subordinate groups which is demanded in the conduct of military operations.

This reconstitution requires the temporary suspension of 'internal' party democracy and the temporary abolition of the principles of democratic centralism which guarantee it. While remaining voluntary and deliberate, more so than ever, party discipline becomes military discipline. Once the situation is analyzed, democratic centralism helps to determine a line and to elect a general staff, after which it should be suspended in order to put the line into effect. The subordinate units go their separate ways and reduce their contact with the leadership to a minimum, according to traditional rules for underground work; in pursuance of the general line they utilize to the best of their ability the greatest margin for initiative granted to them. . . .

The guerrilla movement begins by creating unity within itself around the most urgent military tasks, which have already become political tasks, a unity of non-party elements and of all the parties represented among the *guerrilleros.* The most decisive political choice is membership in the guerrilla forces, in the Armed Forces of Liberation. Thus gradually this small army creates rank-and-file unity among all parties, as it grows and wins its first victories. Eventually, the future People's Army will beget the party of which it is to be, theoretically, the instrument: essentially the party is the army. . . .

The Latin American revolution and its vanguard, the Cuban revolution, have thus made a decisive contribution to international revolutionary experience and to Marxism–Leninism.

Under certain conditions, the political and the military are not separate, but form one organic whole, consisting of the people's army, whose nucleus is the guerrilla army. The vanguard party can exist in the form of the guerrilla foco *itself. The guerrilla force is the party in embryo.*

This is the staggering novelty introduced by the Cuban Revolution.

It is indeed a contribution. One could of course consider this an exceptional situation, the product of a unique combination of circumstances, without further significance. On the contrary, recent developments in countries that are in the vanguard of the armed struggle on the continent confirm and reinforce it. It is reinforced because, whereas the ideology of the Cuban Rebel Army was not Marxist, the ideology of the new guerrilla commands is clearly so, just as the revolution which is their goal is clearly socialist and proletarian. . . .

Thus ends a divorce of several decades' duration between Marxist theory and revolutionary practice. As tentative and tenuous as the reconciliation may appear, it is the guerrilla movement—master of its own political leadership—that embodies it, this handful of men 'with no other alternative but death or victory, at moments when death was a concept a thousand times more real, and victory a myth that only a revolutionary can dream of.' (Che). These men may die, but others will replace them. Risks must be taken. The union of theory and practice is not an inevitability but a battle, and no battle is won in advance. If this union is not achieved there, it will not be achieved anywhere.

The guerrilla force, if it genuinely seeks total political warfare cannot in the long run tolerate any fundamental duality of functions or powers. Che Guevara carries the idea of unity so far that he proposes that the military and political leaders who lead insurrectional struggles in America be 'united, if possible, in one person.' But whether it is an individual, as with Fidel, or collective, the important thing is that the leadership be homogeneous, political and military simultaneously. Career soldiers can, in the process of the people's war, become political leaders (Luis Turcios, for example, had he lived); militant political leaders can become military leaders, learning the art of war by making it (Douglas Bravo, for example). . . .

How can the 'heresy' be justified? What gives the guerrilla movement the right to claim this political responsibility as its own and for itself alone?

The answer is: that class alliance which it alone can achieve, the alliance that will take and administer power, the alliance whose interests are those of socialism—the alliance between workers and peasants. The guerrilla army is a confirmation in action of this alliance; it is the personification of it. When the guerrilla army assumes the prerogatives of political leadership, it is responding to its class content and anticipating tomorrow's dangers. It alone can guarantee that the people's power will not be perverted after victory. If it does not assume the functions of political leadership during the course of emancipation itself, it will not be able to assume them when the war is over. And the bourgeoisie, with all necessary imperialist support, will surely take advantage of the situation.

The guerrilla group's exercise of, or commitment to establish, a political leadership is even more clearly revealed when it organizes its first liberated zone. It then tries out and tests tomorrow's revolutionary measures (as on the Second Front in Oriente): agrarian reform, peasant congresses, levying of taxes, revolutionary tribunals, the discipline of collective life. The liberated zone becomes the prototype and the model for the future state, its administrators the models for future leaders of state. Who but a popular armed force can carry through such socialist 'rehearsals'?. . .

These are the militants of our time, not martyrs, not functionaries, but fighters. Neither creatures of an apparatus nor potentates: at this stage, they themselves are the apparatus. Aggressive men, especially in retreat. Resolute and responsible, each of them knowing the meaning and goal of this armed class struggle through its leaders, fighters like themselves whom they see daily carrying the same packs on their backs, suffering the same blistered feet and the same thirst during a march. The blasé will smile at this vision à la Rousseau. We need not point out here that it is not love of nature nor the pursuit of happiness which brought them to the mountain, but the awareness of a historic necessity. Power is seized and held in the capital, but the road that leads the exploited to it must pass through the countryside. Need we recall that war and military discipline are characterized by rigors unknown to the *Social Contract*?. . .

In most Latin American countries, it is only when the armed struggle has begun or is about to begin that the process of removing the revolution from its ghetto, from the level of academic talk-fests, from a caste of permanent globe-trotters, can get under way. In philosophical language, a certain *problématique* has vanished since the Cuban Revolution, that is to say, a certain way of posing questions which governs the meaning of all possible answers. And it is not the answers that must be changed, but the questions themselves. These 'Marxist-Leninist' fractions or parties operate within the *problématique* which is imposed by the bourgeoisie; instead of transforming it, they have contributed to its firmer entrenchment; they are bogged down in false problems and are accomplices of the opportunistic *problématique*, quarrels over precedence or office-holding in left organizations, electoral fronts, trade union maneuvers, blackmail against their own members. This is what is called quite simply politicking. In order to escape it, there must be a change of terrain, in every sense of the word.

V. SOVIET MARXISM AND A NUCLEAR STRATEGY

Unlike the makers of Western military doctrine, who have been understandably cautious, and even somewhat intimidated by the threats posed by a nuclear war, the Soviet strategists have usually seen such a war as not only practicable but winnable. An exception was Nikita Khrushchev who, during his period of power from the mid-fifties till his overthrow in 1964, saw an atomic war, which would recognize no class distinctions, as culminating in the end of civilized society. Some observers have suggested that this heresy cost the Soviet leader his job. On behalf of what he regarded as Marxist-Leninist orthodoxy, the Chinese communist Lin Piao excoriated Khrushchev as a 'revisionist' for submitting to nuclear blackmail and for having 'no faith in the masses'. (Section VA.)

Both Khrushchev's predecessors and successors, basing their views on the doctrines of Marxism-Leninism, saw a violent conflict between the communist states and the West as the transference of the class struggle to the international stage. (Section VF, G.) Nuclear war was not unthinkable, but given the nature of capitalism, virtually inevitable—again following Clausewitz, the continuation of politics by other means. (Section VB, C.) In the course of such a war, they declared, the morale of the West would give way, and the Soviet defenders of the progressive classes would inevitably triumph over a decadent capitalism. (Section VB, F.) Such an outlook, of course, was in line with the Marxist view of historical development, which saw capitalism as making war necessary, and communism as inevitably triumphant. (See Section VB, D, F, G: also Section III, and Introduction.)

Marshal V. D. Sokolovskii (1897-1968) served as First Deputy Minister of Defence from 1949 to 1960, and Chief of the General Staff of the Soviet Army and Navy from 1952 to 1960. Sokolovskii was the editor of *Soviet Military Strategy*, a volume which represented the collective effort of fifteen

Soviet officers. The work is the first authoritative and systematic presentation of Soviet military doctrine since General A. Svechin, a former Tsarist General who became the first Chief of the Soviet General Staff, published his *Strategy*, in 1926.

In recent years, Soviet military thinkers have mounted a serious effort to apply Marxist dialectics to the science of war. We include one attempt to make use of dialectical concepts such as the 'unity of contradictions' and the 'transition of quantity into quality' in strategical thought. (Section VE.) The author, Colonel S. I. Krupnov, has written a volume on *Dialectics and Military Science*, which was published in Moscow in 1963. The excerpt in this section comes from an article in *Red Star*, Jan. 7 1966. While it may be difficult to see precisely what dialectics have contributed to advance the analysis, a student of strategy can gain some insight into the ways in which Soviet military decisions are articulated by understanding the dialectical component.

Sergei G. Gorshkov (1910-) is the Admiral of the Fleet of the Soviet Union and Commander-in-Chief of the Soviet Navy. For over two decades, he has planned the expansion of a Navy which now rivals that of the Western alliance. In his recent book, *The Sea Power of the State* (1976) Gorshkov attempts to fill the role of a Soviet Mahan, in his efforts to base naval doctrine on the 'study of the experience of past wars . . . on the basis of dialectical materialism.' (See Introductory Remarks to Section I for a note on Byely, and those to Section IV for one on Lin Piao.)

VA. Lin Piao, 'On Revisionists and Nuclear War'*

The fundamental reason why the Khrushchev revisionists are opposed to people's war is that they have no faith in the masses and are afraid of U.S. imperialism, of war, and of revolution. Like all other opportunists, they are blind to the power of the masses and do not believe that the revolutionary people are capable of defeating imperialism. They submit to the nuclear blackmail of the U.S. imperialists and are afraid

* Excerpts from Lin Piao, 'Long Live the Victory of People's War' (1969), in Mallin, ed., *Strategy for Conquest*, pp. 158–61.

that, if the oppressed peoples and nations rise up to fight people's wars or the people of socialist countries repulse U.S. imperialist aggression, U.S. imperialism will become incensed, they themselves will become involved and their fond dream of Soviet-U.S. cooperation to dominate the world will be spoiled. . . .

The Khrushchev revisionists assert that nuclear weapons and strategic rocket units are decisive while conventional forces are insignificant, and that a militia is just a heap of human flesh. For ridiculous reasons such as these, they oppose the mobilization of and reliance on the masses in the socialist countries to get prepared to use people's war against imperialist aggression. They have staked the whole future of their country on nuclear weapons and are engaged in a nuclear gamble with U.S. imperialism, with which they are trying to strike a political deal. Their theory of military strategy is the theory that nuclear weapons decide everything. Their line in army building is the bourgeois line which ignores the human factor and sees only the material factor and which regards technique as everything and politics as nothing. . . .

We know that war brings destruction, sacrifice, and suffering on the people. But the destruction, sacrifice, and suffering will be much greater if no resistance is offered to imperialist armed aggression and the people become willing slaves. The sacrifice of a small number of people in revolutionary wars is repaid by security for whole nations, whole countries, and even the whole of mankind; temporary suffering is repaid by lasting or even perpetual peace and happiness. War can temper the people and push history forward. In this sense, war is a great school. . . .

In diametrical opposition to the Khrushchev revisionists, the Marxist-Leninists and revolutionary people never take a gloomy view of war. Our attitude towards imperialist wars of aggression has always been clear-cut. First, we are against them, and secondly, we are not afraid of them. We will destroy whoever attacks us. As for revolutionary wars waged by the oppressed nations and peoples, so far from opposing them, we invariably give them firm support and active aid. It has been so in the past, it remains so in the present and, when we grow in strength as time goes on, we will give them still more support and aid in the future. It is sheer day-dreaming for anyone to think that, since our revolution has been victorious, our national construction is forging ahead, our national wealth is increasing, and our living conditions are improving, we too will lose our revolutionary fighting will, abandon the cause of world revolution, and discard Marxism–Leninism and proletarian internationalism. Of course, every revolution in a country stems from the demands of its own people. Only when the people in a country are awakened, mobilized, organized, and armed can they overthrow the reactionary rule of imperialism and its lackeys through struggle; their role cannot be replaced or taken over by any people from outside. In this sense, revolution cannot be imported. But this does not exclude mutual sympathy and support on the part of revolutionary peoples in their struggles against the imperialists and their lackeys. Our support and aid to other revolutionary peoples serves precisely to help their self-reliant struggle.

VB. Sokolovskii, 'The Nature of Modern War'*

Marxism–Leninism teaches that war is a socio-historical phenomenon arising at a definite stage in the course of social development. It is an extremely complex social phenomenon, whose essential meaning can be revealed solely by using the only scientific method: Marxist–Leninist dialectics. When discussing the use of Marxist epistemology in the study of war, V. I. Lenin stated that 'dialectics require a comprehensive study of a given social phenomenon as it develops, as well as a study of information which is seemingly extraneous to basic motive forces, to the development of productive forces and to the class struggle.'

Historical experience shows that even the greatest world war, no matter how all-encompassing it may seem, represents only one aspect of social development and completely depends upon the course of that development and upon the political interactions between classes and states. . . .

As is generally known, it was Clausewitz, the German military theoretician, who said: 'War is simply a continuation of

* Excerpts from V. D. Sokolovskii, *Soviet Military Strategy* (Englewood Cliffs, NJ: Rand Corp. and Prentice Hall, 1963), pp. 270 f., 273, 309, 311–14.

politics by other means.' V. I. Lenin, however, introduced a basic correction by adding 'namely, violent' means, which fundamentally altered the statement of the problem. One should emphasize that for Marxist–Leninists, the word 'violence,' when used in a military context, has always meant weapons, the armed forces, and the entire military organization as an instrumentality of war. . . .

Various foreign military publications have recently said that it was wrong to consider war as a continuation of politics with the instruments of violence, and that not only military forces but also various 'non-military' means of conflict—ideological, political, psychological, economic, financial, commercial, diplomatic, scientific, subversive, etc.—must be considered as instruments of war. On this basis they concluded that war is a conflict involving all the instruments of politics, a 'complex' of all the modes and instruments of struggle. Thus, in essence, they equate war, politics, and the class struggle, as a whole, with each other.

The military ideologists of imperialism cannot ignore the fact that a new, nuclear world war initiated by imperialists will inevitably lead to the collapse of capitalism as a social system. Fear for the fate of capitalism and dread of their people, who oppose war, make these ideologists try to justify war, as though it were no longer violent. The British military theoretician, Liddell-Hart, in his book *The Strategy of Indirect Approach*, asserts that instruments of war now not only refer primarily to the armed forces but also to various 'nonmilitary' instruments of conflict: economic pressure, propaganda, diplomacy, subversion, etc. . . .

The Leninist teachings on *the role of the popular masses in war* are of fundamental importance for the correct elucidation of the special features of modern war.

Writing about Tsarism's defeat in the Russo-Japanese War, V. I. Lenin said: 'Wars today are fought by peoples; this brings out more strikingly than ever a great attribute of war, namely, that it opens the eyes of millions to the disparity between the people and the government, which heretofore was evident only to a small class-conscious minority.' In modern wars the disparity between the national interest and the aggressive policy of the imperialistic governments stands out even more clearly.

The masses of the people, depending on their level of political maturity and all the circumstances of the predatory wars conducted by their governments, either passively resist this continuation [of imperialist policy] or struggle actively against it. As a result of the class contradictions which, in Lenin's phrase, tear peoples to pieces in unjust predatory wars, there never has been nor will there be unity within the imperialist states, and [therefore] no chance to pull all the people into support of the war.

The political goals of the just wars of liberation, in defense of a socialist state, are intelligible and dear to the broadest masses, who therefore will conscientiously and actively support and execute their government's policies. Here, the socialist states have an indisputable and reliable advantage over capitalist countries.

A future war will be a clash of two military coalitions with enormous human resources. The socialist coalition has a population of over 1 billion. About 650 million people make up the imperialist blocs. These data show how great a mass of people could be drawn into a third world war. . . .

Experience shows that the large-scale introduction of increasingly complex and highly effective equipment causes increase in numbers of the armed forces generally, as well as of those troops that make use of technical equipment. [This increase takes place] for troops with primary combat missions and also for maintenance units, directorates, staffs, etc. On this basis, Soviet military strategy has concluded that, in spite of the extensive introduction of nuclear weapons and the latest types of different kinds of military equipment, a future world war will require *massive armed forces*.

The armed forces will be of very great size, moreover, because a large number of countries on both sides will be involved in the war and because the geographical scope of the war will be extended. Enormous territories in the deep rear [of the combatant countries] and communications of all types and of tremendous length will have to be protected and defended.

In this connection, one must draw attention to the complete bankruptcy of modern bourgeois theorists who advocate small professional armies with a high level of technical equipment, because they are afraid to arm the masses for class reasons. Similar theories have been advanced in the past. Before World War I, some general staffs, in official documents and military literature as well, tried to prove that, given the increasing power and rate of fire weapons, the forces composed of the already mobilized cadres and reserves and the weapons stocks accumulated in peacetime would be sufficient [to fight the war]. However, as is known, reality upset all these calculations. . . .

If the imperialist bloc initiates a war against the USSR or any other socialist state, it will inevitably become a *world war*, with the majority of the world's countries participating in it.

In its political and social essentials, *a new world war will be the decisive armed collision of two opposing world social systems. This war will inevitably end with the victory of the progressive, communist social and economic system over the reactionary, capitalist social and economic system, which is historically doomed to destruction.* The true balance of political, economic, and military forces of the two systems, which has changed in favor of the socialist camp, guarantees such an outcome of war. However, victory in a future war will not come of itself. It must be thoroughly prepared for and secured in advance. . . .

From the point of view of weapons, a third world war will be a *missile and nuclear war.* The massive use of nuclear weapons, particularly thermonuclear, will make the war unprecedentedly destructive and devastating. Entire states will be wiped off the face of the earth. Missiles carrying nuclear warheads will be the main instruments for attaining the war's aims and for accomplishing the most important strategic and operational missions. Consequently, the leading branch of the armed forces will be the Strategic Missile Forces, and the role and mission of the other branches of the armed forces will be essentially changed. However, final victory will be attained only as a result of the combined efforts of all the branches of the armed forces.

The basic method of waging the war will be by massive missile blows to destroy the aggressor's instruments for nuclear attack and, simultaneously, to destroy and devastate on a large scale the vitally important enemy targets making up his military, political, and economic might, to crush his will to resist, and to attain victory within the shortest possible time.

Under these conditions, the center of gravity of the entire armed struggle will be transferred from the zone of military contact, as in past wars, to deep within the enemy's land, including the remotest places. As a result, the war will be of unprecedented geographic scope.

Since modern weapons permit exceptionally important strategic results to be achieved in the briefest time, both the *initial period of the war* and the methods of breaking up the opponent's aggressive plans by dealing him in good time a crushing blow will be of *decisive significance for the outcome of the entire war.* Hence, the main task of Soviet military strategy is working out means for reliably *repelling a surprise nuclear attack by an aggressor.*

VC. Byely, 'Nuclear War and Clausewitz'*

Bourgeois ideologists intensify their attacks against the Marxist–Leninits definition of war as a continuation of politics by violent means. These attacks take mainly one of two forms. One part of the bourgeois ideologists eulogises Clausewitz as 'a great classicist' whose theories are applicable to all times, extols his merits in every way, calls his book *On War* an unsurpassed military-theoretical 'bible' and thereby distorts historical truth. . . . Bourgeois ideologists aver that there is nothing new in the Marxist–Leninist teaching on war and that it has been fully and wholly drawn from Clausewitz, a representative of bourgeois military-theoretical thought.

In extolling Clausewitz and ignoring historical experience, the ideologists of the reactionary bourgeoisie, especially those closely connected with the top brass of the aggressive NATO bloc, make it appear that no changes have taken place in the interrelation between politics and war. They justify the policy of nuclear blackmail, insist on keeping thermonuclear war in their political arsenal, advocate the thermonuclear and conventional arms race, and close their eyes to the danger of a new world war.

H. Kahn, an ideologist of US imperialism, who has been named the 'Clausewitz of the nuclear age', develops in his

* Excerpts from Byely *et al., Marxism–Leninism on War and Army* (1972), pp. 40–4, 46.

books the idea of the 'admissibility' of thermonuclear war as a political instrument. He says that 'war is a terrible thing, but so is peace', believes that after a third world war with its use of weapons of mass destruction, with its colossal destruction and enormous toll of victims there will be . . . 'normal and happy lives for the majority of survivors and their descendants.' . . .

Other bourgeois ideologists, realising that a thermonuclear war will be fatal to capitalism, have fallen into the other extreme, and declare that the former view on the interrelation between politics and war is outdated and has lost all significance. These ideologists endeavour to prove that nuclear missile weapons have consigned the formula that war is a continuation of politics by violent means to history. . . .

The main argument against the definition of war as a continuation of politics by violent means builds on the fact that nuclear war actually abolishes the distinction between front and rear and threatens both belligerents with catastrophic consequences. Undeniably, these arguments of Western sociologists and writers on military matters, holding different philosophical views and standing on different political positions, contain 'an iota of truth'. This shows that they are aware of the enormous danger constituted by nuclear war as an instrument of aggressive imperialist policies. Yet, despite all that their arguments are one-sided and untenable.

This is because, firstly, in criticising Clausewitz's theory and the formula that war is a continuation of politics by violent menas, the bourgeois writers offer no solution for the problem of the interrelations between politics and war themselves, do not help to clear up the problem, but only confuse it.

Secondly, bourgeois sociologists and writers on military subjects use the pretext that the formula of war being a continuation of politics by violent means is outdated as a basis for their attempts to discredit the most important component of the Marxist–Leninist teaching on war and politics, and aver that it is inapplicable in the nuclear age. This is the latest variant in the many attempts to refute the Marxist–Leninist view on politics and war, on the interrelation between the two, a variant which they, for reasons of camouflage, sometimes try to pass off as love of peace. . . .

Marxist-Leninist methodology makes it possible to solve the question of the interrelation between politics and armed force in the possible nuclear war in a consistently scientific way. As regards its essence, such a war would also be a continuation of the politics of classes and states by violent means. Politics will determine when the armed struggle is to be started and what means are to be employed. Nuclear war cannot emerge from nowhere, out of a vacuum, by itself, without the deliberately malicious politics of imperialism's most aggressive circles. As the First and Second World Wars, which were the products of the aggressive, predatory policies of the imperialist states, as also the numerous limited, local wars, unleashed by the imperialists after 1945, a nuclear missile war, if it is allowed to come to a head, will also be a product of the aggressive policies of US imperialism and its partners in various blocs.

The social, class content of nuclear missile war and its aims will be determined by politics. The new world war will be, on one side, the continuation, weapon and instrument of criminal imperialist policies being implemented with nuclear missiles. On the other side, it will be the lawful and just counteraction to aggression, the natural right and sacred duty of progressive mankind to destroy imperialism, its bitterest enemy, the source of destructive wars.

Hence, the nuclear missile war will also be a continuation of politics, although some ideologists of imperialism deny this; in fact, it will be even more 'political'. In his remarks to Clausewitz's book *On War* Lenin stressed the idea that 'war seems the more "warlike", the more political it is. . . .' This emphasises the growth in scope and depth of the influence politics exercises on war, expresses a certain regularity—the 'politisation' of war in step with its industrialisation and mechanisation. Armed struggle with the use of nuclear missiles and other weapons will ultimately be subordinated to the interests of a definite policy, will become a means of attaining definite political aims. . . .

In the new war, if it should be allowed to happen, victory will be with the countries of the world socialist system which are defending progressive, ascending tendencies in social development, have at their command all the latest kinds of weapons, and enjoy the support of the working people of all countries. The balance of forces between the two systems, the logic of history, its objective laws, prescribing that the new in social development is invincible—all this predicts such an outcome. The might of the Soviet state, of the entire socialist community, which possesses the economic, moral-political and military-technical preconditions for utterly routing any aggressor, substantiates this view. Other factors and forces which will inevitably spring into action as soon as war breaks out must also not be thrown off the scales; they will include decisive anti-imperialist actions by the people, political, diplomatic, international legal, ideological and other actions against those responsible for unleashing a nuclear adventure.

VD. Sokolovskii, 'Limited War'*

Reactionary scientists in various disciplines—sociologists, economists, and military theoreticians—who reflect an imperialist aspiration to world domination, develop various theories and doctrines in military strategy. In the pages of the bourgeois press, we see flashing by as in a kaleidoscope: 'brinkmanship,' 'the strategy of massive retaliation,' 'the strategy of deterrence,' 'graduated strategy,' 'doctrine of containment,' 'doctrine of liberation'; and recently, since the United States' loss of its nuclear monopoly, particular interest in so-called limited or small wars has arisen in many capitalist countries.

The appearance of a theory of limited war is not accidental. Observing the colossal success of the Soviet Union and other socialist countries in economic development, science, technology, and culture, the imperialists began to be convinced not only of the impossibility of crushing the socialist system, but also of the fact that a new world war would inevitably be disastrous for capitalism. However, the achievement of political aims in capitalist society is inconceivable without war. The military theoreticians of imperialism scurry about in search of solutions of military and political problems which, on one hand, would avoid the destruction of the capitalist system, and on the other hand, would lead to the realization

* Excerpts from Sokolovskii, *Soviet Military Strategy* (1963), pp. 136 f.

of expansionist aims. Limited war, in the opinion of American military theoreticians, is most responsive to these aims. In advocating the theory of limited war, American strategists thus try to keep the United States safe from retaliatory nuclear strikes, to suppress movements of national liberation, to preserve the colonial system, and to create additional stimuli for its economy in order to extract maximum profits.

In the imperialist plans, limited war is also particularly important as a pretext for starting wars against the socialist countries.

Bourgeois strategy is reactionary in its social and political aims since it serves the interests of imperialist aggressors, who conduct unjust and predatory wars in order to seize foreign territories, to suppress national liberation movements, and to enslave the people of other countries.

Bourgeois military strategy is reactionary, not only in its political content, but in its ideological, theoretical and philosophical bases as well, because it appraises social phenomena, including war, by means of an anti-scientific bourgeois sociology and an idealistic and metaphysical philosophy.

The military strategy of imperialist states is intended to preserve and to extend [the life of] the capitalist system, which has outlived itself, to preserve the rotten system of colonialism, and to combat the most advanced and most progressive system of human society, the socialist system.

VE. Krupnov, 'Dialectics and Military Science'*

All the phenomena of nature, society, and thought have inherent internal contradictions. Precisely these contradictions are the source of all development. Therefore, the most important condition for the proper understanding of all of the processes of the world, V. I. Lenin taught, is 'the understanding of them as a unity of contradictions.'

The phenomenon of armed conflict is not an exception to this general rule. On the contrary, war is contradictory throughout. It arises from socio-economic and political antag-

* Excerpts from Colonel S. I. Krupnov, 'According to the Laws of Dialectics', *Red Star*, Jan. 7 1966. [In W. R. Kintner and H. F. Scott, *The Nuclear Revolution in Soviet Military Affairs* (Norman, Okla.: University of Oklahoma Press, 1968), pp. 238–42.]

onisms between classes, governments, and nations, and represents a degree of the highest aggravation of the contradictions, the sharpest form of their settlement. Therefore, only a *correct understanding of the nature of the social conflict which has evoked the war and realization of its political aims make it possible to determine with the greatest exactness the military-strategic nature of the armed conflict.*

The basic contradiction of the modern era is the contradiction between the two social systems–socialism and imperialism. And, naturally, if the imperialists unleash thermonuclear war, it will inevitably become a world war, a coalition war, and it will have an exceptionally violent and decisive nature. It will inevitably be marked by the final victory of the forces of socialism over the forces of imperialism. But wars can also be caused by other contradictions: between capitalistic monopolies and workers, between the metropolis and the colonies, between imperialist powers themselves. In this case, armed conflict might have a different nature.

Thus, the knowledge of social conflicts and of the political goals of the war makes it possible to foresee its nature. But such knowledge alone is not enough to determine with sufficient certainty all the diversity of those methods and uses which will be used by soldiers on the battlefield. For this, it is necessary to understand the *contradiction between weapons, military equipment, and methods and forms of armed conflict* which always exist in military affairs. This contradiction is explained by the fact that the material base, forces, and means of waging war change more quickly than methods and forms of conflict. Between them arises a disparity. Sooner or later it is detected, and people must eliminate it. It was thus, for example, after the appearance of firearms and after the invention and introduction of tanks and airplanes.

The contradiction between the means and forms of armed conflict in our time has acquired special acuteness. At first it seemed to some people that nuclear rocket weapons would not bring in any qualitative changes to the organization and direction of troops and in the methods of their actions. But tests of the new weapons and research of their possibilities convincingly showed that they were unconventional and different in principle than weapons of the past. The search was begun for new organizational forms and principles of waging armed conflict.

The problem is not limited to the search for the most effective way of using modern weapons. The appearance of new means of struggle always brings into being corresponding *countermeans*, which in the end also lead to changes of the methods of military operations. The 'struggle' of tanks and antitank means, submarines and antisubmarine means, airplanes and antiairplane defense, radio-means and means of radio jamming, rockets and antirockets—this is the axis around which revolves the development of military affairs, including the development of methods and forms of armed conflict.

Or this contradiction. Since war began to be waged, armies have always had to attack or defend themselves. *Attack and defense* are two contrasting kinds of military action. But it is the kind of contrast which organically ties and depends on each other and the correct understanding of the development of each of them is possible only by examining attack and defense in close connection with each other.

In present-day war with the use of the latest means of attack, just as it was earlier, only attack can lead to the defeat of the enemy and victory over him. But even in such a war, one cannot manage without defense. It is another matter that *now the nature of both attack and defense has essentially changed and the tendency to* rapprochement *is observed* of these basic aspects of combat actions. A strategic nuclear rocket strike, for example, *combines* in itself, simultaneously, the function of attack and defense.

Since ancient times one of the principles of military art has been the concentration of force on the main direction of military actions. This principle preserves its significance in present-day war also. But now, both on the march, in attack, and in defense, troops must act in dispersed groupings in order not to be convenient targets for strikes with nuclear weapons. At the same time they must remain constantly strong, able to carry strikes to the enemy at any moment.

Thus, still another most acute contradiction arises—the *contradiction between concentration and dispersion.* Every kind of improvement in troop mobility is the chief form of solving this contradiction.

Present-day combat actions are distinguished by high maneuverability, waged on a wide front and at exceptionally high tempos. Such a nature of armed conflict significantly complicates the control of troops. Now the commander must make a decision and convey it to his subordinates in the shortest period of time. At the same time the quantity and the difficulty of questions to be decided by the military leader have increased. This contradiction is overcome by the method of seeking *new ways of control* based on the widest use of electronic computer machines and small mechanizations. These devices, of course, cannot replace the commander. Today, he, as never before, must have deep and all-round knowledge, extremely developed intuition, the ability for logical thinking, mathematical methods of knowledge, and high moral qualities.

A decisive influence on the development of the principles of systems of control of troops is rendered by the constant existence of *contradiction between their centralization and decentralization.* The use of the nuclear rocket weapon and the swiftest use of the results of its strike is unthinkable without strict centralization of control. At the same time military actions will be spread over a large area without set fronts and with great gaps between combat formations. This demands concessions of independence to commanders of subunits, units, and groups, which are significantly greater than in past wars.

Thus, contradictions and the overcoming of them are the vital source of the development of methods and forms of armed combat and of all military affairs. To notice, in time, emerging contradictions and to determine the proper course of their solution means to find the key to solving problems which are standing before military science and before the theoreticians and practitioners of military affairs.

The revolution in military affairs evoked by the appearance of the new weapon has not been received by everyone in the same way. Some have affirmed that the nuclear weapon is allegedly absolute and that it completely negates massive land armies and air and naval fleets. Others have supposed that the changes in military affairs must be gradual for, they say, the nuclear rocket weapon is no different in principle from the old, and will not bring in great changes in the methods and forms of armed conflict but will only add a few features to it.

These different points of view reflect the age-old question: How does the process of development of methods and forms of armed conflict proceed—gradually and smoothly, or by leaps in a revolutionary manner?

The key to the correct understanding of the problem is given by dialectical-materialism. It teaches that *the development of military affairs, as all development, is subject to the actions of the law of the transformation of quantitative changes to qualitative ones.* New weapons lead to qualitative changes of methods and forms of armed conflict, not at once, but only at the time when its quantity reaches a significant size.

VF. Byely, 'War and Ideology'*

Ideology fulfils the function of a specific instrument of war. Ideological means of struggle are specific because, on the whole, they influence the course and results of military operations and the war not directly, but through the impact they make on the minds of the people, on their world outlook, views, morale and fighting efficiency. Ideological means are able to strengthen the morale of the troops and of the population of one's own country, and to erode the morale and political principles of the army and the population of the enemy countries. . . .

The ideological struggle and ideology in general have played different roles in wars fought in different historical periods. In the past their role was limited above all as regards their influence on the enemy. In the 20th century, when the technical possibilities of influencing the masses have grown, when the masses have become more enlightened and are drawn ever deeper into politics, the role of the ideological struggle in war has greatly increased. In just wars the spread of communist ideology plays an enormous role in ensuring the victories of the working masses over their enemies.

In modern conditions the ideological struggle preceding war and attending it is particularly sharp, and defeat in war is

* Excerpts from Byely, *Marxism–Leninism on War and Army* (1972), pp. 57 ff., 61–4, 66 f.

not only a military, economic and political defeat, but also an ideological one. Nowadays a war cannot be begun and conducted, let alone won, without a thorough ideological preparation of the people and the army. . . .

In the epoch of feudalism, . . . religious ideology was dominant. All annexationist, predatory wars, and also the revolutionary wars the peasant masses waged against the feudal lords, were conducted under the banner of religious ideas. But while the form—religious ideology—was similar, the political aspirations underlying this ideology differed.

With the advent of capitalism and bourgeois national states, political ideology became decisive in the wars waged by these states and the bourgeoisie often counterposed political ideology to the religious ideology of the feudals and the clergy.

Typical of the period of the progressive development of capitalism were wars aimed at resolving questions of bourgeois-democratic transformations, at overthrowing foreign oppression and defending national freedom During that epoch bourgeois ideology was mainly a national ideology, used as an instrument in the struggle for the setting up of bourgeois national states with a national culture of their own.

This ideology had a progressive role to play. It was the spiritual power that helped the bourgeoisie rally the popular masses round it. The national ideology continues to play this relatively progressive role at definite stages of the national liberation struggle of the peoples in the colonial and dependent countries against imperialist oppression.

The national ideology created in the epoch of national wars made a deep imprint on the petty bourgeoisie and on a definite part of the proletariat. It has been used by the bourgeoisie in the predatory wars of the imperialist period. By using the 'national' ideology and speculating on the 'defence of motherland' concept, the imperialist bourgeoisie deceived the people in the First World War.

After the Second World War the 'national' ideology was no longer able to meet imperialist interests. This is because that ideology does not unite, but disunites the imperialist states according to the national principle and hampers the establishment of unity within their aggressive military blocs. . . .

It was only in the civil wars of the past that different

ideologies opposed each other. This was the case in the wars of slaves against slave-owners, of the serfs against the landowners, and in the wars of the proletariat against the bourgeoisie. As we said above, the participants in peasant wars formally adopted a religious ideology, but in political content it differed radically from the ideology of the feudal lords.

Modern wars are generally clashes between opposing ideologies. Two ideologies opposed each other in the war of the first socialist state against the foreign interventionists and the internal counter-revolutionaries, in the war against nazi Germany, and in the wars of the peoples of Korea, Vietnam and Cuba against the imperialist aggressors. In the wars of the colonial peoples for their independence, progressive national ideology opposes the reactionary ideology of imperialism. . . .

The assertion that modern wars are ideological ones is particularly absurd because ideological contradictions have never been and never can be primary: they have always been and always will be secondary, derivative of economic contradictions.

This applies also to the epoch of religious wars, to which the bourgeois ideologists like to refer as examples of ideological wars. In reality religious wars were an upshot of economic causes and pursued very definite political, class aims. Religious views were not the cause of these wars, they were but ideological weapons.

All talk of the modern bourgeois ideologists about the epoch of ideological wars is directed against the basic Marxist-Leninist principle that war is the continuation of the policies of a class by violent means, and that politics itself is 'a concentrated expression of the economy'. The aim of this talk is to make it appear as though the presence of opposing ideologies in the two world systems is the source of a possible third world war, as though communist ideology contains the seeds of war.

The former British Minister Michael Stuart [Stewart] believes that the Soviet Union's refusal to discontinue the ideological struggle prevents the establishment of good-neighbourly relations between countries and peoples. . . .

In the modern world a violent struggle is going on between the two ideologies—communist and bourgeois. This struggle is the reflection in the people's mind of the historical transition from capitalism to socialism. An important problem in this struggle is the issue of war and peace and the different attitudes adopted to it in the socialist and in the imperialist camps.

Communism brings eternal peace to mankind. The most important content of communist ideology is internationalism, humanism, love of peace, the mutual assistance of peoples in all spheres of social life. The fighters for communism are inspired by the noble idea of emancipating mankind from exploitation and their actions are directed at imbuing the minds of people with the idea that wars are inadmissible. But, as long as there is a danger of war, there must also be a consistent and irreconcilable struggle against the military ideology of imperialism. . . .

Communist ideology is superior not only to the avowedly reactionary bourgeois theories, but also to various pacifist views. Rejecting all wars and insisting on general conciliation, irrespective of the class positions of the sides, pacifism disarms the working people—it is not an idea that can exercise a deep and enduring influence. The pacifists' appeal to religion, to the Church, does not make pacifism any more convincing. . . .

Communist ideology is permeated with optimism, based on scientific prevision. It rejects the pessimistic bourgeois ideology in all its forms, and expresses the inevitable triumph of the forces of progress over the dark forces of reaction.

VG. Byely, 'Wars between Opposing Social Systems'*

The US monopoly bourgeoisie constantly inculcates the peoples with the idea that a world war against the USSR and the whole socialist camp is inevitable. . . .

But imperialism is unable to recover the historical initiative it has lost, or to reverse the modern world developments. It is quite obvious that the reactionary political aims of the imperialists are adventuristic. They contradict the objective laws of social development. Therefore the nuclear war imperialism is planning against the socialist community with the aim of stopping the forward march of history will be regressive as

* Excerpts from Byely, *Marxism-Leninism on War and Army* (1972), pp. 99 f., 102 f., 142, 392 f.

concerns its social role and most reactionary as regards its political content. On the part of the peoples of the socialist states and of progressive mankind as a whole, it will be a holy war for freedom and independence, a just liberation war. Such a world war will be a violent and tense struggle between opposing social forces, a class war on an international scale.

Because of this sharply pronounced class character the political and military aims of the sides at war will be decisive and the use of nuclear weapons will lend it an unprecedentedly destructive character. A thermonuclear war would kill hundreds of millions of people, lay waste entire countries, inflict irretrievable losses to material and spiritual culture. Mankind would be thrown back for many decades. . . .

Only the enemies of socialism can stupidly insist on an 'export' of revolution, on an encroachment by world socialism by means of force on the 'free institutions' of the capitalist world. Revolution is not made to order but ripens in the process of historical development and breaks out at moments conditioned by a whole complex of internal and external factors.

War is not an essential element in that complex, is not the decisive condition for revolution, there is no simple and direct link between war and revolution. Imperialist wars do not always lead to revolution and not every revolution is preceded by a war. Yet, war and revolution are not isolated political phenomena. There is a definite connection between them. This connection manifested itself most clearly in the First and Second World Wars, which exerted a major impact on the revolutionary process.

World war exacerbates the internal and external contradictions of capitalism, erodes the state apparatus of the bourgeoisie and gives rise to a deep political crisis of the whole system of imperialism. War raises the people's political awareness, creates the conditions in which the working people rise to struggle against the bourgeois system. The trials of war and the heavy toll of human lives the unjust war exacts objectively impel the people to revolution. Lenin meant this when in 1917 he said that world war inevitably leads to revolution. . . .

Should a world nuclear war be unleashed against the will of the masses, the latter will have to decide a task of historic importance and to use different means for its implementation. This task will be the destruction of the entire system of capitalism, which cannot exist without wars, just as it cannot exist without class and national oppression. The fact that the above-mentioned regularities will act with even greater force in the event of a nuclear war postulates as a certainty that the working people will refuse to put up any further with a system breeding wars.

Let us review the basic ideas of Soviet military doctrine.

As regards its socio-political nature, the future war, should the imperialists succeed in unleashing it, will be a bitter armed clash between two diametrically opposed social systems, a struggle between two coalitions, the socialist and the imperialist, in which every side will pursue the most decisive aims.

As regards the means used, this war may be a nuclear one. Even though nuclear weapons will play the decisive role in the war, final victory over the aggressor can be achieved only as a result of the joint actions of all the arms of the services, which must utilise in full measure the results of the nuclear strikes at the enemy and fulfil their specific tasks.

As regards its scope the nuclear war will be a world war and an inter-continental one. This is determined both by its socio-political content and by the fact that both sides possess missiles of practically unlimited range, atomic missile-carrying submarines, and strategic bombers. The war will engulf practically the entire planet.

It will be waged by methods differing radically from those used in the past. Formerly the direct aim of all military actions was to rout the enemy's forces, without which it was impossible to reach his vital strategic centres. Now the situation has changed. The use of nuclear missile weapons makes it possible to attain decisive military results in a very short time, at any distance and on vast territories. In the event of war not only groupings of the enemy's armed forces will be subjected to destructive nuclear strikes, but also his industrial and political centres, communication centres, everything that feeds the arteries of war.

The first massive nuclear strikes are able largely to predetermine the subsequent course of the war and to inflict such heavy losses in the rear and among the troops that they may place the people and the country in an extraordinarily difficult position.

Nevertheless, troops possessing an adamant will for victory and inspired by the lofty aims of a just war, can and must wage active offensive operations with whatever forces have survived and strive to rout the enemy completely.

Soviet military doctrine proceeds from the assumption that the imperialists are preparing a surprise nuclear attack against the USSR and other socialist countries. At the same time they consider the possibility of waging military operations with conventional weapons and the possibility of these operations escalating into military actions involving the use of nuclear missile weapons. Therefore, the chief and main task of the Armed Forces consists in being constantly ready to repel a sudden attack of the enemy in any form, to foil his criminal intentions, no matter what means he might use.

VH. Gorshkov, 'The Navy and Nuclear Strategy'*

The scientific, ideological and theoretical basis of the building of the armed forces of our State is the Marxist-Leninist theory of war and the army. . . . Unlike many authorities of the past who confine the content of military science simply to the sphere of military art, Vladimir Il'ich regarded the theory and practice of the business of war as an inseparable part of the social activity of people living in a class society. As far back as 1905 in an article *Fall of Port Arthur* he showed the effect of the objective patterns of modern war, the decisive role in it of the popular masses, the significance of moral and economic factors and concluded that the outcome of armed struggle depends not only on the army but also on the whole people, i.e. on the rear (in the widest sense of the word). . . . In the epoch of imperialism when wars are waged by peoples this tenet assumes special importance. Just wars generate patriotism, the high morale of the people and army and, conversely, unjust wars cannot produce in them a high morale since they are waged in the interests of the greed of the exploiters. . . .

* Excerpts from S. G. Gorshkov, *The Sea Power of the State* (Annapolis, Md.: Naval Institute Press, 1979), pp. 130 f., 168, 213, 247 f., 279, 284. [Originally published in 1976.]

Perusal of the content of the military doctrines of the imperialist states shows that whatever their name they are all aimed against the world socialist system and their principal task is to save capitalism which is doomed by history.

According to the theories of the ideologists of imperialism, the only means of saving capitalism is military force. At present, in their view, it can only be nuclear strike forces which in the post-war period have become the main argument used by the aggressive military doctrines of the chief imperialist countries. Among these forces a growing role is being played by the navy. . . .

Naval art is a historical category, since each period of history has its own theory and practice of armed conflict at sea suitably reflecting the point reached in the development of material means for such conflict.

In the course of the centuries-old history of navies, naval art has developed unevenly. It has known smooth, gradual movements ahead and tempestuous surges, raising it to a height previously appearing unattainable. Periods of decline mostly coincided with a strengthening of reaction and the stagnation of economic and political life. Flourishing periods usually corresponded to revolutionary events in the life of nations. . . .

Naval art, like any other scientific theory, is intimately connected with practice, and rests on the lessons from past wars. . . . Without study of the experience of past wars and its critical application, the development of naval art cannot be ensured. Study of historical experience on the basis of dialectical materialism is a method of grasping the patterns of armed struggle at sea, the laws, lines and directions of the development of naval art. . . .

Policy, as Lenin taught, is a concentrated expression of the economy, the state of which primarily determines the power of such an important instrument of policy as are the armed forces of the nation. It is precisely in the state of the armed forces of a given country that its economic power is reflected.

Graphic confirmation of this and a conventional indicator of the level of development of the economy of a country may be the navy. . . .

To build a modern warship, a high level of development of

all branches of industry and science of the country is needed. The building of an individual ship meeting modern requirements is possible only with the widest co-operation, only if each of the branches of industry connected with shipbuilding supplies products of the highest quality. As a rule, several hundred establishments take part in the building of a fighting ship. The creation of a fleet as a whole, sufficient in complement to solve the tasks facing it with all the means of supply for its normal service, is possible only for states with a powerful economy.

The long time taken to develop the material-technical resources of a fleet, the relatively short service life for ships and the attendant danger of morale decay of the forces of the fleet make special demands on science, which must lay down the guidelines for building a fleet for years and even decades ahead.

The navy, as a constituent part of the armed forces of the state, has a further distinctive feature, namely the ability to demonstrate graphically the real fighting power of one's state in the international arena. This feature is usually utilized by the political leadership of the imperialist countries to frighten off potential adversaries. It should be noted that the arsenal of the means for such displays, used by the diplomacy of these countries, is constantly expanding.

As is known, in the last few years it has become common to hold displays of missile weapons, combat aviation and various military equipment on an international scale, pursuing as well as a commercial, another aim: to surprise potential enemies with the perfection of this equipment, exert on them a demoralizing influence by the power of one's weapons even in peacetime, instil in them in advance the idea that efforts to combat aggression are futile. This technique has often been employed throughout the history of military rivalry. True, such a propaganda technique far from always reaches the goals set, primarily because the means of war displayed impress the viewer merely as a potential force. The navy is another matter. Ships appearing directly offshore represent a real threat of actions, the time and ways of realizing which are determined by their command. And if such a threat was quite great in the past, it has now considerably grown since modern ships are carriers of nuclear missile weapons and aircraft, the zone of reach of which may extend to the whole territory of a state.

Demonstrative actions by the fleet in many cases have made it possible to achieve political ends without resorting to armed struggle, merely by putting on pressure with one's own potential might and threatening to start military operations.

Thus, the fleet has always been an instrument of the policy of states, an important aid to diplomacy in peacetime. To this corresponded the very nature of a navy, the properties peculiar to it, namely, constant high combat readiness, mobility and ability in a short time to concentrate its forces in selected areas of the ocean. In addition, the neutrality of the waters of the World Ocean means that the forces of fleets can be moved forward and concentrated without violating the principles of international law and without providing the other side with formal grounds for protests or other forms of counteraction....

Scientific and technical progress in the military realm has brought forward new criteria for determining the real fighting power of each of the branches of the armed forces, the principal one being the ability to use most rationally such a decisive resource of armed struggle as nuclear missile weapons. Therefore, forces possessing nuclear missile strategic weapons of intercontinental range have come to the fore.

Scientific and technical progress has produced submarines as the most perfect carrier of modern weapons, the launching site of which is in effect the whole World Ocean. The fleet concentrates in itself numerous mobile carriers of strategic weapons, each of which may carry a very large number of long-range missiles and is capable of manœvring with launching sites over an area exceeding many times the area which land-based missile troops can use. Sea carriers of strategic means also possess the ability to manœvre in depth, sheltering themselves by width of water and using it not only for protection but also for masking, which greatly adds to the viability of naval strategic weapons systems. Thus, objective conditions of armed conflict in a nuclear war produce as a strike nuclear missile force the missile-carrying fleet, rationally combining the latest achievements of science and technology, enormous strike power and mobility, viability of strategic means and high readiness for their immediate use....

The Party teaches that as long as there persists imperialism, the aggressive nature of which has not changed, a real danger of the outbreak of a new world war remains. In the leading capitalist states there is no slackening of preparations for the material-technical base for war, military budgets are growing, and new arms systems, above all, the latest submarine nuclear missile systems are being actively created.

All this has determined the need and rationale of the efforts which are being made in our country to develop the navy—the basic component of the sea power of the state capable of withstanding the oceanic strategy of imperialism.

INDEX

Cont

Truth is concrete → War is War

Prod. Yonnes